ALABAMA

:: OTHER BOOKS IN THE BEST TENT CAMPING SERIES

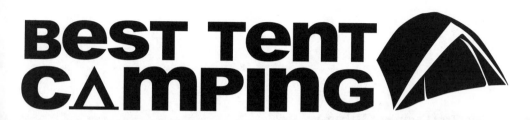

BEST TENT CAMPING
ALABAMA

YOUR CAR-CAMPING GUIDE TO SCENIC BEAUTY, THE SOUNDS OF NATURE, AND AN ESCAPE FROM CIVILIZATION

JOE CUHAJ

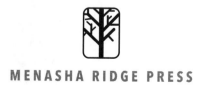

MENASHA RIDGE PRESS

Best Tent Camping: Alabama

Copyright © 2013 by Joe Cuhaj
All rights reserved
Printed in the United States of America
Published by Menasha Ridge Press
Distributed by Publishers Group West
First edition, first printing

Library of Congress Cataloging-in-Publication Data

Cuhaj, Joe.
   Best tent camping, Alabama : your car-camping guide to scenic beauty, the sounds of
nature, and an escape from civilization / Joe Cuhaj.
      pages cm
   ISBN 978-0-89732-574-5 — ISBN 0-89732-574-5; eISBN 978-0-89732-948-4
   1. Camp sites, facilities, etc.—Alabama—Guidebooks. 2. Camping—Alabama—Guidebooks.
   3. Automobile travel—Alabama—Guidebooks. 4. Alabama—Guidebooks. I. Title.
   GV191.42.A2C85 2013
   796.5409761—dc23
                              2013003868

Cover design by Scott McGrew
Cover photos by Joe Cuhaj
Text design by Annie Long
Cartography by Steve Jones and Joe Cuhaj
Indexing by Rich Carlson

MENASHA RIDGE PRESS
P.O. Box 43673
Birmingham, Alabama 35243
menasharidge.com

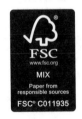

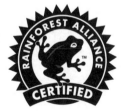

CONTENTS

● ●

:: METRO REGION

:: MOUNTAIN REGION

BEST CAMPGROUNDS

• •

ACKNOWLEDGMENTS

I cannot possibly thank all of the people who made this book possible in the short space allotted for such things. Countless people chimed in with suggestions for campgrounds and why they thought their choice should be included in this book. I took all to heart and used many. Thanks to all of you for your input.

There are a few people, however, to whom I need to extend special thanks, because without them the pages you now hold in your hand would not have been possible. Topping the list are Susan Haynes and Amber Kaye Henderson with Menasha Ridge Press. Susan believed in this project and got the ball rolling. Amber had the tough job of making sense of my scribblings and hieroglyphics. Thanks to both of you.

For input and guidance on campgrounds to visit, I have to thank Jim Felder and Fred Couch with the Alabama Scenic River Trail, Rob Grant with the Alabama Department of Economic and Community Affairs, Grey Brennan and his staff at the Alabama Tourism Department, and Lesley Hodge with the US Forest Service.

I would be remiss if I didn't acknowledge the many US Army Corps of Engineers volunteer campground hosts and US Forest Service park attendants for their generosity in sharing information. Always eager to impart knowledge of their campground and region, they added a new depth to many entries.

And finally, and most importantly, I have to thank my wife, Maggie. She was with me—literally—every step of the way. Even when I had no leg to stand on, she was there to help me with the research for this book. I could not have done this without you.

PREFACE

Picture this: Buchanan, New York, 1963. A young man, and by *young* I mean 5 years old, joins his family on the first day of what would become a family tradition—camping on a beautiful strip of beach along the banks of the Hudson River. Yes, *the* Hudson River. We were oblivious to the environmental struggles this majestic river was and would be facing. All we knew was that the river provided one long endless summer of fun with swimming, water skiing, hiking, and, of course, camping.

We spent many hot summer nights in that behemoth of a tent we lugged along with us, a giant Coleman canvas cabin structure with massive aluminum poles that took hours to erect, but once up hosted many late-night gin rummy games and endless conversations around lantern light.

And that's where it started, and for the life of me, I can't remember a time when I was not in camping mode, whether it was pitching a tent along a beautiful hiking trail, beside a scenic river, or in a public campground, the tent was always at the ready to rekindle those memories and make new ones.

Eventually I married my wife, Maggie, and we moved from New Jersey to her hometown of Mobile, Alabama, along the state's Gulf Coast. Quickly I learned that Alabama has some of the most beautiful public campgrounds anywhere. They're much more than just a place to put up a tent for a night or two. They are scenic, inviting, friendly, and teeming with recreational opportunities, and in Alabama the adventures seem endless. I have car camped on crisp winter nights at DeSoto State Park when the campground was nearly deserted and snow silently fell

around me; I have spent nights at Monte Sano State Park and left the warm glow of my campfire to take in planetarium shows and glimpses of the heavens through the telescopes at the Von Braun Astronomical Observatory before turning in for the night; and I have spent more than one night along the banks of Lake Chinnabee in the Talladega National Forest, using it as a base camp for amazing hikes to high mountain peaks, ridges, and cascading waterfalls.

Recreational opportunities and amazing landscapes abound at or near Alabama's campgrounds. Fishermen have plenty of opportunities to try for some world-record fishing along the banks of thousands of miles of rivers and waterways and, of course, on the Gulf of Mexico. You can explore deep caves with massive stalagmites and magical underground rivers; hike to cascading waterfalls; spend hours bird-watching or admiring wildflowers; play historian with a trip back in time to historic Civil War battlefields, ancient Native American mounds, and towns that are all but memories; or canoe and kayak meandering blackwater rivers or Class III, IV, or V whitewater rapids. And that's only the start.

The number and types of flora and fauna in Alabama keep botanists and zoologists up at night. Some of the most rare and beautiful wildflowers bloom here, wildlife range from wild turkey to black bear to the American alligator, and when it comes to fish, the state's thousands of miles of rivers, lakes, and streams are home to more than 144 species—more than the entire state of California has. I guess one statistic sums the state up nicely—Alabama is the fifth-most ecologically diverse state in the country.

Camping in Alabama lets you experience this diversity first hand. You can camp beneath a rock shelter in a beautiful, deep canyon with glowing insects called dismalites that illuminate the rock walls; pitch your tent atop the state's highest mountain, Cheaha, for spectacular views; settle in for a night along the banks of the second-largest river delta in the country; or sleep under the stars at the site of the last major battle of the Civil War.

As for the organization of the book, I've divided the state into the four regions defined by the Alabama Tourism Department. The first is the Metropolitan, or Metro, Region. Located just above the middle of the state, it includes Birmingham, Tuscaloosa, and Anniston. Here you will find spectacular mountain camping in the Talladega National Forest, as well as plenty of outings in historical state parks.

Next there is the Mountain Region, which is located in the northern quarter of the state and includes the cities of Huntsville, Florence, and Fort Payne. Not only will you experience mountains here but canyons as well, such as in the Sipsey Wilderness of the Bankhead National Forest and the deepest canyon east of the Mississippi, Little River Canyon, near Fort Payne.

The River Region includes the state capital, Montgomery, as well as Auburn, Dothan, and some smaller but remarkable historical towns on the state's west side. The region gets its name from the myriad

of waterways crisscrossing this area as they meander southward to the Gulf of Mexico. And I mean a myriad! Take a look at the state seal and you will see this tapestry of rivers, and that's only a small fraction.

Finally we have the Gulf Region, which includes the city of Mobile plus Baldwin, Escambia, and Monroe Counties. Although its coastal miles are minimal compared with, say, those of Florida or Texas, Alabama still has some of the prettiest beaches you'll find anywhere, fantastic resort-type camping, and beautiful campgrounds along some of the major rivers flowing into the Gulf of Mexico.

The most common question with a book like this is about my selection process for the 50 campgrounds. My primary goal was to make this guide a sample of the many wonderful campsites the state has to offer and to provide a little something for everyone. Whether you're a beginning or veteran camper, whether or not you have children, or whether you want to use your campground as a base to explore historical towns or beautiful landscapes, I think that you'll find a campsite just right for you. I hope that you'll find a good cross section of camping experiences so that you can visit the landscapes and people that make camping in Alabama so special.

But the campgrounds you read about here are just the beginning. There are hundreds more for you to visit, all equally impressive. I hope that this book inspires you to go out and find your own special campground in Alabama where you'll make memories for yourself and your family.

INTRODUCTION

● ●

How to Use This Guidebook

The **publishers** of Menasha Ridge Press welcome you to *Best Tent Camping: Alabama.* Whether you're new to this activity or you've been sleeping in your portable outdoor shelter over decades of outdoor adventures, please review the following information. It explains how we have worked with the author to organize this book and how you can make the best use of it.

Some passages in this introduction are applicable to all of the books in the *Best Tent Camping* guidebook series. Where this isn't the case, such as in the descriptions of weather, wildlife, and plants, the author has provided information specific to your state.

THE RATINGS & RATING CATEGORIES

As with all of the state-by-state books in the publisher's *Best Tent Camping* series, this guidebook's author personally experienced dozens of campgrounds and campsites to select the top 50 locations in this state. Within that universe of 50 sites, the author then ranked each one in the six categories described below. As a tough grader, the author awarded few five-star ratings, but each campground in this guidebook is superlative in its own way. For example, a site may be rated only one star in one category but perhaps five stars in another category. This rating system allows you to choose your destination based on the attributes that are most important to you.

★ ★ ★ ★ ★ The site is **ideal** in that category.

★ ★ ★ ★ The site is **exemplary** in that category.

★ ★ ★ The site is **very good** in that category.

★ ★ The site is **above average** in that category.

★ The site is **acceptable** in that category.

Beauty

Beauty, of course, is in the eye of the beholder, but panoramic views or proximity to a lake or river earn especially high marks. A campground that blends in well with the environment scores well, as do areas with remarkable wildlife or geology. Well-kept vegetation and nicely laid-out sites also up the ratings.

Privacy

The number of sites in a campground, the amount of screening between them, and physical distance from one another are decisive factors for the privacy ratings. Other considerations include the presence of nearby trails or day-use areas, as well as proximity to a town or city that would invite regular day-use traffic and perhaps compromise privacy.

Spaciousness

The size of the tent spot, its proximity to other tent spots, and whether or not it is defined or bordered from activity areas are the key consideration. The highest ratings go to sites that allow the tent-camper to comfortably spread out without overlapping neighboring sites, or picnic, cooking, or parking areas.

Quiet

Criteria for this rating include several touchstones: the author's experience at the site, the nearness of roads, the proximity of towns and cities, the probable number of RVs, the likelihood of noisy ATVs or boats, and whether a campground host is available or willing to enforce the quiet hours. Of course, one set of noisy neighbors can deflate a five-star rating into a one-star (or no-star), so the latter criterion—campground enforcement—was particularly important in the author's evaluation of this category.

Security

How you determine a campground's security will depend on who you view as the greater risk: other people or the wilderness. The more remote the campground, the less likely you are to run into opportunistic crime, but the more remote the campground, the harder it is to get help in case of an accident or dangerous wildlife confrontation. Ratings in this category take into consideration whether there was a campground host or resident park ranger, proximity of other campers' sites, how much day traffic the campground received, how close the campground was to a town or city, and whether there was cell-phone reception or some type of pay phone or emergency call button.

Cleanliness

A campground's appearance often depends on who was there right before you and how your visit coincides with the maintenance schedule. In general, higher marks went to those campgrounds with hosts who cleaned up regularly. The rare case of odor-free toilets also gleaned high marks. At campgrounds without a host, criteria included trash receptacles and evidence that sites were cleared and that signs and buildings were kept repaired. Markdowns for the campground were not given for a single visitor's garbage left at a site, but old trash in the shrubbery and along trails, indicating infrequent cleaning, did secure low ratings.

THE OVERVIEW MAP & KEY

Use the overview map on the inside front cover to pinpoint the location of each campground. The campground's number follows it throughout this guidebook: from the overview map, to the map key facing the overview map, to the table of contents, and to the profile's first page. A map legend that details the symbols found on the campground-layout maps appears on the inside back cover.

CAMPGROUND-LAYOUT MAPS

Each profile contains a detailed map of campground sites, internal roads, facilities, and other key items.

CAMPGROUND ENTRANCE GPS COORDINATES

All 50 of the profiles in this guidebook include a box showing the GPS coordinates for each site entrance. The intersection of the latitude (north) and longitude (west) coordinates orients you to the entrance. Please note that this guidebook uses the degree–decimal minute format for presenting the GPS coordinates. Example:

GPS COORDINATES   N32° 58.693'   W85° 13.272'

To convert GPS coordinates from degrees, minutes, and seconds to the above degrees–decimal minutes format, the seconds are divided by 60. For more on GPS technology, visit **usgs.gov.**

WEATHER

The weather in Alabama is as distinctive as its environment. Along the Gulf Coast you'll experience a subtropical climate, while to the north cold and snowy winters are common. But of course, weather isn't that cut-and-dried.

Average temperatures in the north range from 46°F in January to 80°F in July. On the coast the temperatures range from 52°F in the winter to 85°F in summer. Yes, the coast does experience cold snaps of below 30°F in the winter, sometimes even below zero, but they're usually short-lived and last only a day or two.

Overall the weather across the state makes it a pleasure to camp out any time of the year, but there are a few caveats. Being in a subtropical environment you can expect extended days of high heat and humidity throughout the summer. This makes for a deadly combination and a heat index that easily soars over 100° many days throughout the summer.

Alabama is particularly prone to a couple of big weather issues in the summer. Because of the heat and humidity, the state experiences extremely dangerous pop-up summertime thunderstorms. These squalls can drop 2 or more inches of rain in less than an hour and be accompanied by dangerous lightning and, in the north, tornadoes.

The other is hurricane season, which generally falls between May and November. Even though Alabama has a relatively small strip of land along the Gulf of Mexico, the area has seen devastating storms in the last decade, including Ivan, Dennis, and, of course, Katrina. And even though a hurricane afflicts the most wind and water damage along the coast, areas hundreds of miles away can still feel its effects. As a matter of fact, most injuries and deaths resulting from a hurricane occur well inland from flooding. Be sure to check for severe weather updates with the National Weather Service and local news outlets regularly during the summer, no matter what part of the state you travel.

FIRST-AID KIT

A useful first-aid kit may contain more items than you might think necessary. These are just the basics. Prepackaged kits in waterproof bags (Atwater Carey and Adventure Medical make them) are available. As a preventive measure, always take along sunscreen and insect repellent. Even though quite a few items are listed here, they pack down into a small space.

- Ace bandages or Spenco joint wraps
- Adhesive bandages, such as Band-Aids
- Antibiotic ointment *(Neosporin or the generic equivalent)*
- Antiseptic or disinfectant, such as Betadine or hydrogen peroxide
- Aspirin, acetaminophen *(Tylenol)*, or ibuprofen *(Advil)*
- Benadryl or the generic equivalent, diphenhydramine *(in case of allergic reactions)*
- Butterfly-closure bandages
- Emergency poncho
- Epinephrine in a prefilled syringe *(for severe allergic reactions to bee stings and so on)*
- Gauze *(one roll and six 4-by-4-inch compress pads)*
- LED flashlight or headlamp
- Matches or pocket lighter
- Mirror for signaling passing aircraft
- Moleskin/Spenco 2nd Skin
- Pocketknife or multipurpose tool
- Waterproof first-aid tape
- Whistle *(it's more effective in signaling rescuers than your voice)*

FLORA & FAUNA PRECAUTIONS

Poisonous Plants

Poison ivy and poison sumac thrive across the Southeast. Some people have reactions to these plants while others don't. Your best bet is to not take the chance and avoid them by learning how to identify them.

Ever hear the old adage "leaves of three, let it be"? Poison ivy can be either a thick vine clinging to trees or a ground cover. The plant is easily identifiable by its three leaflets.

If you happen upon a poison sumac tree in the forest, you might think that it would look very nice as an ornamental plant in your home—don't go there! The tree itself grows 25–30 feet tall, has a 5-inch-diameter trunk, is covered with broad leaves with each leaf containing 7–13 leaflets, and is adorned with groupings of small white berries that birds love. Sumac is found in wet marshes, forests, and swamps, and because of this, the plant is found only in the lower two-thirds of the state and is virtually nonexistent from the Mountain Region north.

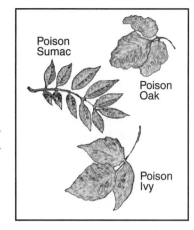

What makes these plants so irritating is the oil in their sap, called urushiol. Usually within 12–14 hours after contact, a rash begins to develop with raised lines, sometimes blisters, and a terrible itch.

If you have these symptoms, don't scratch the infected area. Wash and dry the rash thoroughly, then apply calamine lotion or a similar product that will help dry it. If itching or blistering is severe, seek medical attention. And remember, oil-contaminated clothes, pets, or hiking gear can easily cause an irritating rash on you or someone else, so wash not only any exposed parts of your body but also clothes, gear, and pets.

Mosquitoes and Yellow Flies

You can't escape them. They can be found everywhere from north to south Alabama. Mosquitoes are literally after your blood, and while it's rare, they can infect humans with the West Nile virus. Culex mosquitoes, the primary variety that can transmit West Nile virus, thrive in urban rather than natural areas. They lay their eggs in stagnant water and can breed in any standing water that remains for more than five days. Most people infected with West Nile virus have no symptoms, but some may become ill, usually 3–15 days after being bitten.

Anytime you expect mosquitoes to be buzzing around, you may want to wear protective clothing, such as long sleeves, long pants, and socks. Loose-fitting, light-colored clothing is best. Spray clothing with insect repellent. Remember to follow the instructions on the repellent and to take extra care to protect children against these insects.

Another nuisance in the South is yellow flies. These yellow-bodied insects live in shady, humid areas along the edges of rivers, creeks, streams, and forests. Like the mosquito, yellow flies are out for a little blood, and once one bites you, expect the crew to join in. You could find yourself with 20 or 30 yellow flies attacking at one time.

Unlike the mosquito their bite is fierce. While they can bite any part of the body, they mainly focus on the head, neck, and shoulders, and once they have your scent, they are almost impossible to get rid of. The best way to avoid them is to stay in sunny open areas. If you are on the move, for example hiking, move at a fast jog. And unfortunately, insect repellents have little effect on yellow flies.

Snakes

More than 50 species of snakes call Alabama home, but only 6 are venomous (poisonous): the copperhead, eastern diamondback rattler, eastern cottonmouth or water moccasin, pygmy rattlesnake, and timber rattlesnake. Most of these are common throughout the state with the exception of the pygmy rattlesnake and eastern diamondback, which are described as being rare to uncommon and are believed to be declining in numbers. In any event a good rule of thumb is to give whatever animal you encounter a wide berth and leave it alone.

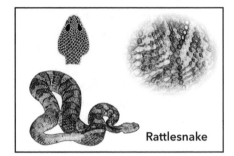

Copperhead

Rattlesnake

Alligators

Nothing adds to your camping adventure like spotting an alligator or two relaxing in the sun or floating along a river or bayou. Alligators can be found from the Gulf to Montgomery. Remember, alligators are naturally afraid of humans, but don't feed them! Feeding them changes the pecking order, and they become reliant on people for food, and that could mean you or your dog.

Ticks

Ticks like to hang out in the brush that grows along trails, and while there are certain species of ticks that live in one region of the state or another, it is safe to say that ticks are common throughout Alabama.

Warm weather brings them out. Ticks are not insects but arachnids that need a host to continue their life cycle. The primary types of ticks are deer and dog ticks and are very small when they light upon you. It usually takes several hours for a tick to attach itself and transmit any diseases. The best strategy when you're in the woods is to do a tick check every half hour or so, that is, visual inspections to make sure that you don't have any unwanted hitchhikers on board. Do another check at camp and then again when you take a shower; be sure to check your entire body.

Ticks that haven't latched on are easily removed but not easily killed. If you find one in the woods, it's best to simply toss it aside. If you find one on your person, in the bathroom, you can flush it down the toilet. For ticks that have embedded, removal with tweezers is best.

CAMPGROUND ETIQUETTE

Here are a few tips on how to create good vibes with fellow campers and wildlife you encounter.

- Make sure that you check in, pay your fee, and mark your site as directed. Don't make the mistake of grabbing a seemingly empty site that looks more appealing than your site. It could be reserved. If you're unhappy with the site you've selected, check with the campground host for other options.

- Be sensitive to the ground beneath you. Place all garbage in designated receptacles or pack it out if none is available. No one likes to see the trash that someone else has left behind.

- It's common for animals to wander through campsites, where they may be accustomed to the presence of humans (and our food). An unannounced approach, a sudden movement, or a loud noise startles most animals. A surprised animal can be dangerous to you, to others, and to themselves. Give them plenty of space.

- Plan ahead. Know your equipment, your ability, and the area where you are camping—and prepare accordingly. Be self-sufficient at all times; carry necessary supplies for changes in weather or other conditions. A well-executed trip is a satisfaction to you and to others.

- Be courteous to other campers, hikers, bikers, and anyone else you encounter.

- Strictly follow the campground's rules regarding the building of fires. Never burn trash. Trash smoke smells horrible, and trash debris in a fire pit or grill is unsightly.

- Everyone likes a fire, but bringing your own firewood from home is now frowned upon by most campground operators. Bringing in wood from out of the area could introduce pests that are harmful to the forest. Use deadfall found near your campsite or purchase wood at the camp store.

HAPPY CAMPING

There's nothing worse than a bad camping trip, especially because it's so easy to have a great time. To assist with making your outing a happy one, here are some pointers:

- Reserve your site in advance, especially if it's a weekend or a holiday, or if the campground is wildly popular. Many prime campgrounds require at least a six-month lead time on reservations. Check before you go.

- Pick your camping buddies wisely. A family trip is pretty straightforward, but you may want to reconsider including grumpy Uncle Fred, who doesn't like bugs, sunshine, or marshmallows. After you know who's going, make sure that everyone is on the same page regarding expectations of difficulty (amenities or the lack thereof, physical exertion, and so on), sleeping arrangements, and food requirements.

- Don't duplicate equipment, such as cooking pots and lanterns, among campers in your party. Carry what you need to have a good time, but don't turn the trip into a cross-country moving experience.

- Dress for the season. Educate yourself on the temperature highs and lows of the specific part of the state you plan to visit. It may be warm at night in the summer in your backyard, but up in the mountains it will be quite chilly.

- Pitch your tent on a level surface, preferably one covered with leaves, pine straw, or grass. Use a tarp or specially designed footprint to thwart ground moisture and to protect the tent floor. Do a little site maintenance, such as picking up the small rocks and sticks that can damage your tent floor and make sleep uncomfortable. If you have a separate tent rain fly but don't think you'll need it, keep it rolled up at the base of the tent in case it starts raining at midnight.

- Consider taking a sleeping pad if the ground makes you uncomfortable. Choose a pad that is full-length and thicker than you think you might need. This will not only keep your hips from aching on hard ground, but it will also help keep you warm. A wide range of thin, light, or inflatable pads is available at camping stores today, and these are a much better choice than home air mattresses, which conduct heat away from the body and tend to deflate during the night.

- If you are not hiking in to a primitive campsite, there is no real need to skimp on food due to weight. Plan tasty meals and bring everything you will need to prepare, cook, eat, and clean up.

- If you tend to use the bathroom multiple times at night, you should plan ahead. Leaving a warm sleeping bag and stumbling around in the dark to find the restroom—whether it be a pit toilet, a fully plumbed comfort station, or just the woods—is not fun. Keep a flashlight and any other accoutrements you may need by the tent door and know exactly where to head in the dark.

- Standing dead trees and storm-damaged living trees can pose a real hazard to tent campers (foresters call these widow-makers for obvious reasons.) These trees may have loose or broken limbs that could fall at any time. When choosing a campsite or even just a spot to rest during a hike, look up.

A WORD ABOUT BACKCOUNTRY CAMPING

Following these guidelines will increase your chances for a pleasant, safe, and low-impact interaction with nature.

- Adhere to the adages "Pack it in; pack it out" and "Take only pictures; leave only footprints." Practice "leave no trace" camping ethics while in the backcountry.

- In Alabama, open fires are permitted except during dry times when the US Forest Service may issue a fire ban. Backpacking stoves are strongly encouraged.

■ Hang food away from bears and other animals to prevent them from being introduced to (and becoming dependent on) human food. Yes, Alabama has bears. A growing number of black bears, as a matter of fact. Wildlife learns to associate backpacks and backpackers with easy food sources, thereby influencing its behavior.

■ Bury solid human waste in a hole at least 3 inches deep and at least 200 feet away from trails and water sources; a trowel is basic backpacking equipment. More and more often, however, the practice of burying human waste is being banned. Using a portable latrine (which comes in various incarnations, basically a glorified plastic bag, given out by park rangers) may seem unthinkable at first, but it's really no big deal. Just bring an extra-large zip-top bag for extra insurance against structural failures.

VENTURING AWAY FROM THE CAMPGROUND

If you go for a hike, bike ride, or other excursion into the wilderness, here are some precautions to keep in mind.

■ Always carry food and water, whether you are planning to go overnight or not. Food will give you energy, help keep you warm, and sustain you in an emergency until help arrives. Bring potable water or treat water by boiling or filtering before drinking from a lake or stream.

■ Stay on designated trails. Most hikers get lost when they leave the trail. Even on the most clearly marked trails, there is usually a point where you have to stop and consider which direction to head. If you become disoriented, don't panic. As soon as you think you may be off-track, stop, assess your current direction, and then retrace your steps back to the point where you went awry. If you have absolutely no idea how to continue, return to the trailhead the way you came in. Should you become completely lost and have no idea of how to return to the trailhead, remaining in place along the trail and waiting for help is most often the best option for adults and always the best option for children.

■ Be especially careful when crossing streams. Whether you are fording the stream or crossing on a log, make every step count. If you have any doubt about maintaining your balance on a log, go ahead and ford the stream instead. When fording a stream, use a trekking pole or stout stick for balance and face upstream as you cross. If a stream seems too deep to ford, turn back. Whatever is on the other side is not worth risking your life.

■ Be careful at overlooks. Although these areas may provide spectacular views, they are potentially hazardous. Stay back from the edge of outcrops and be absolutely sure of your footing: a misstep can mean a nasty and possibly fatal fall.

■ Know the symptoms of hypothermia. Shivering and forgetfulness are the two most common indicators of this insidious killer. Hypothermia can occur at any elevation, even in the summer. Wearing cotton clothing puts you especially at risk, because cotton, when wet, wicks heat away from the body. To prevent hypothermia, dress in layers using synthetic clothing for insulation, use a cap and gloves to reduce heat loss, and protect yourself with waterproof, breathable sleeping bag.

■ Take along your brain. A cool, calculating mind is the single-most important piece of equipment you'll ever need in the woods. Think before you act. Watch your step. Plan ahead. Avoiding accidents before they happen is the best recipe for a rewarding and relaxing camping trip.

Metro Region

1

Amity Campground

"Spectacular sunrises over shimmering waters"

Deep within the mixed oak-and-pine forests and fertile rolling farmlands of southeast Alabama, on the banks of the Chattahoochee River directly on the Georgia state line, you'll find yet another one of the state's amazing US Army Corps of Engineers sites, Amity Campground.

The Chattahoochee River begins its journey to the Gulf of Mexico in the Blue Ridge Mountains of north Georgia. The river finally reaches Alabama here at West Point Lake and forms the border between the two states the remainder of its journey south. Amity Campground, on the southern end of the lake, is the northernmost Corps of Engineers campground on the Alabama side of the river.

Like Walter F. George and George W. Andrews Lakes farther south, West Point Lake was created by impounding the river. In 1962 Congress directed the Corps of Engineers to build West Point Dam to control flooding, provide a navigable water route to the gulf, develop and encourage wildlife and fish habitats, and provide hydroelectric power to the region. The dam is 7,250 feet long and creates a lake with a surface area of 25,900 acres and a shoreline of 525 miles.

:: Ratings

BEAUTY: ★ ★ ★ ★
PRIVACY: ★ ★ ★
SPACIOUSNESS: ★ ★ ★
QUIET: ★ ★ ★ ★
SECURITY: ★ ★ ★ ★ ★
CLEANLINESS: ★ ★ ★ ★

The power plant here generates enough electricity each year to run 24,000 homes. The dam was closed to tourists immediately after the attacks of 9/11 but has recently reopened. Tours must be scheduled in advance and have a minimum of 10 people. Contact West Point Dam at 706-645-2937 for more information.

As for the campground, the bulk of it juts into the lake, offering spectacular sunrises over the shimmering waters. This is a birding paradise, with many rare and beautiful species calling the lake, and campground, home. It is not uncommon to see an eagle or osprey soaring high overhead or to catch a glimpse of the rare great cormorants. Other birds you may see include king rails, greater white-fronted geese, gulls, purple gallinules, and, in the winter, several thousand species of migratory birds.

Once again, Amity Campground and the surrounding lake are an angler's dream, especially if you're a bass fisher. Largemouth and spotted bass are the main catches, but you can also try your hand at catfish, crappie, and bream. There are two cement boat ramps for you to launch from, along with plenty of room for bank fishing. And don't forget to bring along that Alabama freshwater-fishing license.

There is no shortage of activities. Besides fishing, the campground has a playground and basketball, tennis, and volleyball courts.

You'll find two nice hiking trails here as well. One is a 0.5-mile interpretive trail

:: Key Information

ADDRESS: 1001 County Road 393, Lanett, AL 36863

OPERATED BY: US Army Corps of Engineers

CONTACT: 334-499-2404; reservations 877-444-6777; tinyurl.com/amitycamp

OPEN: March–September

SITES: 96

SITE AMENITIES: Gravel pad, picnic table, grill, fire ring, lantern post, water, power

ASSIGNMENT: First-come, first-serve or by reservation

REGISTRATION: At entry gate or by reservation

FACILITIES: Flush toilets, hot showers, laundry, playground, lake swimming, fishing, fish-cleaning station, basketball court, volleyball court

PARKING: At each site; additional parking inside Mill Run, River Forest, and Pine Bluff Loops across from campsites

FEE: Improved, $24; primitive, $16

ELEVATION: 689'

RESTRICTIONS:

■ **Pets:** On leash only; not allowed in beach areas, playgrounds, or restrooms

■ **Fires:** In fire ring or grill only; use only deadfall

■ **Alcohol:** Prohibited

■ **Vehicles:** 4/site

■ **Other:** Quiet hours 10 p.m.–6 a.m.; 8 people/site; must obtain pass and display in windshield before entering; gate locked 10 p.m.–7 a.m.; 14-day stay limit

(be sure to pick up a booklet from the park attendant, so you can identify trees and wildlife), and the other is a 0.4-mile boardwalk to a beaver pond, where you will see waterfowl and other wildlife atop the observation platform.

Of the 96 sites at Amity, numbers 63–73 are tent-only with a gravel pad and fire ring. Here you will find some of the most beautiful views of the lake on sites 65–73. All others are improved with electricity, water, a fire ring, grill, a picnic table, and lantern post. The tent sites are compact crushed gravel pads. Many are waterfront, but if you can get them, shoot for numbers 37–62. These sit on a peninsula that juts into the lake and have wonderful views and cool lake breezes.

Clean and spacious restrooms, along with two bathhouses, each large enough for the number of campers, are scattered throughout the campgrounds. The men's and women's section have two hot showers that are handicap-accessible, and the facilities are heated. Plus, the bathhouses are cleaned twice daily.

And as we have come to expect at Corps of Engineers campsites, security is excellent with a locking gate after-hours, park attendant station, and camp hosts who live next to the gate.

Make a note about the time zone difference here. While most of Alabama is in the Central Time Zone, several towns bordering Georgia, including Lanett, use Eastern Time.

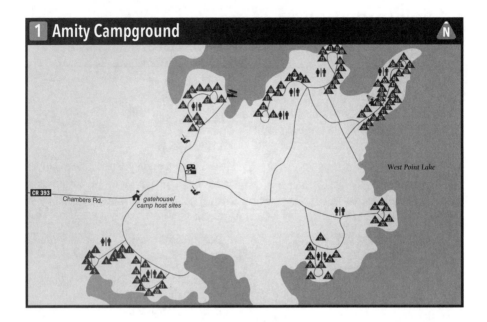

:: Getting There

From Lanett travel north 1 mile on South State Line Road. The road turns into County Road 212. Continue traveling an additional 6.1 miles and turn right onto CR 393. The park entrance will be to the right.

GPS COORDINATES N32° 58.693' W85° 13.272'

2

Brierfield Ironworks Historical State Park

"Brierfield is far from crowds, providing a beautiful, tranquil oasis with a backdrop of more than 150 years of history."

The **centerpiece** of Brierfield Ironworks Historical State Park is the furnace itself, named Bibb for the county where it was constructed. The story of the Bibb Furnace begins in 1862, when Caswell Campbell Huckabee saw the region's commercial potential. Working with several partners, Huckabee formed the Bibb County Iron Company. Built with slave labor, the furnace was soon producing what was described as "the toughest and most suitable iron for making guns above any other in the South."

The Confederacy bought the foundry in 1863 for the price of $600,000 and nine slaves. Not long after that, the Union Army took notice and came to town, burning everything in its path, including the furnace.

In later years individuals would try to resurrect the Bibb Furnace. The former chief of ordnance for the Confederacy, Josiah Gorgas, assembled a crew to make the furnace operational once again, but the effort did not succeed for long, and in 1873 the furnace's flames died out for a second time.

The history of the Bibb Furnace didn't end there, however. In 1882 a man named Thomas Jefferson Peter and a group of investors brought the furnace back online one last time. It became very profitable, so much so that the town of Brierfield became known as the Magic City of Bibb County. In 10 years, however, the magic disappeared. Birmingham's new and modern metal furnaces could produce 10 times as much iron as Bibb, which forced the foundry out of business again, this time for good.

That's where the story could have ended, but the Bibb County Historical Society urged officials to establish a park here: Brierfield Ironworks Historical State Park.

Through the society's efforts, Brierfield lives once again. Nestled deep in the woods on 45 acres, Brierfield is far from crowds, providing a beautiful, tranquil oasis with a backdrop of more than 150 years of history.

While smaller than neighboring Tannehill (see page 43), the park still does an excellent job of keeping the history alive. The big furnace was toppled by the Union Army, and much was lost to the elements, and even lost to scavengers seeking souvenirs. A shelter now protects the crumpled remains of the brickwork. Quietly stroll around the structure and you can almost

:: Ratings

BEAUTY: ★ ★ ★ ★
PRIVACY: ★ ★ ★
SPACIOUSNESS: ★ ★
QUIET: ★ ★ ★ ★
SECURITY: ★ ★ ★ ★
CLEANLINESS: ★ ★ ★ ★

:: Key Information

ADDRESS: 240 Furnace Pkwy., Brierfield, AL 35035	**FACILITIES:** Flush toilets, hot showers, playground, pool, camp store
OPERATED BY: Alabama Historic Commission	**PARKING:** At each site
CONTACT: 205-665-1856; brierfieldironworks.com	**FEE:** Improved (for 4 people), $20; primitive (for 4 people), $12; add $3 for each additional person
OPEN: Year-round	**ELEVATION:** 437'
SITES: 25 improved, 9 primitive	**RESTRICTIONS:**
SITE AMENITIES: Improved–picnic table, fire ring with grill, water, power; primitive–picnic table, fire ring	■ **Pets:** On leash only
	■ **Fires:** In fire ring only
ASSIGNMENT: First-come, first-serve	■ **Alcohol:** Prohibited
	■ **Vehicles:** 2/site
REGISTRATION: Pay attendant at camp store	■ **Other:** Quiet hours 10 p.m.–6 a.m.; 1 tent (4 people)/site

see the history, imagining the thick, black smoke billowing from a 60-foot smokestack and hundreds of men toiling in the heat to make the desperately needed iron for the war effort. A nice hiking trail leads to the top of a hill overlooking the ruins.

Today, Brierfield has grown, covering more than 1,500 acres. There are 25 improved campsites, each with power, water, a picnic table, and a fire ring. Improved sites 1–10 are more suited for RVs than tent campers. The sites are well separated, providing some privacy. Sites 18–22 are located along a small creek, Furnace Creek, which has a nice flow in the spring. Site 11 is located near the remains of the furnace, giving you a historic view to wake up to.

The park is rimmed with nine primitive sites. Tucked away in the hardwood forest are two very nondescript ones, which are on the very north side of the park just across the road from the main campground. The remainder are found in an open field between the main gate and furnace. Each primitive site has a picnic table and a fire ring as well as simple dirt or grass pad.

The park has a swimming pool by the bathhouse. If you register for an improved site, the pool is free; otherwise a pool pass is $5 per person.

The camp store, located in the office, has a good selection of items and plenty of snacks. A very clean bathhouse with hot showers is outside the campground at the south end of the park. The shower doors are made from old-fashioned wooden planks, reminiscent of days gone by.

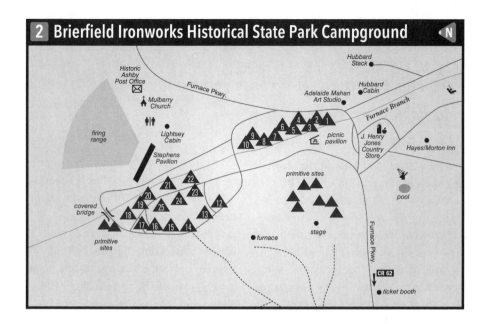

:: Getting There

From McCalla take AL 25 South 6.6 miles. Turn left onto County Road 62. Travel 0.4 mile and take the first left onto CR 62/Furnace Parkway. In 0.3 mile arrive at the park entrance.

GPS COORDINATES   N33° 02.290'   W86° 56.931'

3

Cheaha State Park

"The perfect place to set up base camp and explore remarkable landscapes"

Saying that **Cheaha State Park** is a standout in the Alabama State Park system is not an overstatement. The park is located atop Cheaha Mountain, the state's tallest at 2,407 feet (Cheaha comes from the Creek word *chaha,* meaning "high place.")

Located within the 390,000-acre Talladega National Forest, in the east-central part of the state, Cheaha is the perfect place to set up base camp and explore remarkable waterfalls and beautiful mountain vistas; swim in deep, cold mountain stream pools; and simply admire nature.

As with many Alabama state parks, Cheaha was built by the Civilian Conservation Corps in the 1930s. The CCC was created during the Great Depression under the orders of President Franklin Roosevelt. Its simple mission: create thousands of jobs for able but unemployed young men through an array of public works projects ranging in scope and size from dams to roadways to state parks.

The centerpiece of Cheaha is a signature piece of CCC engineering, a massive stone fire tower at the summit built entirely by hand with stone mined from the region. A CCC museum was just opened within the tower in spring 2013.

Hiking is Cheaha's prime draw. The handicap-accessible Boardwalk Trail offers a 1-mile trek out to Bald Rock and a spectacular view of the surrounding Talladega Mountains. The park's second trail is for the more adventurous. The Rock Garden Trail begins at the base of the mountain and climbs to the top with a steep elevation gain. You'll often find rock climbers scaling cliffs and rappelling here.

And the surrounding Talladega National Forest, with hundreds of miles of trails, is just a short drive, or walk, from Cheaha. A few outstanding routes include the Chinnabee Silent Trail, which travels alongside beautiful rushing streams, waterfalls, and gorges; the Cave Creek Trail through tunnels of bright rhododendrons in the spring and more magnificent views; and the world-famous Pinhoti Trail. The Pinhoti travels more than 130 miles, the entire length of the forest, and then into Georgia, where it connects to the Appalachian Trail. The Pinhoti provides a wide variety of loop hikes for day hikers.

Cheaha State Park is also a prime gathering spot for fall-leaf spotters. Thousands of people flock to the mountain late October–late November to see the spectacle provided by the north-Alabama hardwoods.

:: Ratings

BEAUTY: ★ ★ ★ ★ ★ ★
PRIVACY: ★ ★ ★ ★
SPACIOUSNESS: ★ ★ ★ ★
QUIET: ★ ★ ★ ★
SECURITY: ★ ★ ★ ★
CLEANLINESS: ★ ★ ★ ★

:: Key Information

ADDRESS: 19644 AL 281, Delta, AL 36258

OPERATED BY: Alabama State Parks

CONTACT: 256-488-5111; 800-610-5801; alapark.com/cheaharesort

OPEN: Year-round

SITES: Mountain Top (43 improved), Cheaha Lake (30 improved), Picnic Trail (25 primitive), CCC (30 primitive)

SITE AMENITIES: Improved—picnic table, fire ring, grill, water, power; Primitive—picnic table, fire ring, grill

ASSIGNMENT: First-come, first-serve or by reservation

REGISTRATION: Pay attendant at office or by reservation

FACILITIES: Flush toilets, hot showers, playground, pay phone, pool, restaurant, camp store

PARKING: At each site

FEE: Improved, $22 ($3 additional fee on Saturday–Sunday and holidays); primitive, $16

ELEVATION: 2,213'

RESTRICTIONS:

■ **Pets:** On 6-foot leash only

■ **Fires:** In fire ring only

■ **Alcohol:** Permitted

■ **Vehicles:** 2/site

■ **Other:** Quiet hours 10 p.m.–6 a.m.

Needless to say, Cheaha is a very popular campground and will be full most of the year except in the very dead of winter, late December and early January. Summertime and the weekend of the Talladega 500 NASCAR race is when the park is most packed, followed closely by the fall, when leaf seekers descend on the area.

You'll find four campgrounds in the park. A semiprimitive one sits along what is known as the Picnic Trail and is located across the road from the stone CCC fire tower. The 25 nondescript sites here are simple grassy plots, some a bit rockier than others. Each has a fire ring and a picnic table. The large field sports a decent view to the west, though a few sites along the edge of the area slope down considerably. There are several sites along the picnic area at the top of the mountain. These spots give you a good view of the surrounding mountains to the west, but radio and television antennas across the road to the east, next to the fire tower, detract from the view. Additionally, these campsites are right up against the road

so evening traffic could be a nuisance. Community water spigots are available in this campground.

The second campground is Mountain Top (also called the Upper Campground). While the sites are a bit close together, they aren't close enough to take away from your camping pleasure. The pads are light-packed gravel, and all sites include water, power, a picnic table, a fire ring, and a grill.

The two bathhouses in the loop are exceptional. Hand-built by the CCC, these stone structures house clean restrooms and hot showers. Best of all, they have excellent heating if you find yourself on the mountain on a frosty winter morning. There isn't really a best site in this campground. Each one is exceptional with plenty of shade. The thick forest obscures any views. If you have kids or don't like walks to the bathhouses on cold mornings, then your best bets are sites 3, 8, 14, 16, 19, 21, 23, or 25, which are each adjacent to one of the two bathhouses.

The final two campgrounds are not in the main state park but down the hillside

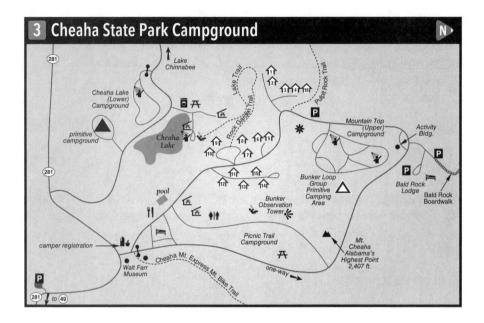

on a side road just off of AL 281. The Lower Campground is popular with folks who want to be near Cheaha Lake (the lake is across the road from the campground). There are 30 sites in the Lower Campground, all with power, water, picnic tables, and fire rings. The campsite has its own coded entry gate, which is closed 24 hours a day.

The Primitive Campground, which was the original CCC campground and just reopened spring 2013, was Cheaha's first campground. Each of the 30 sites has a fire ring, and a community water spigot is available. The campground has restrooms, but the closest bathhouse is in the Cheaha Lake (Lower) Campground.

Whichever campground you choose, you'll either register at the country store or reserve by phone. When you arrive, visit the country store and get a code to enter the gated area of the park or the Cheaha Lake (Lower) Campground. And speaking of the country store, it has a pretty good selection of supplies in case you forgot to pack something.

For a diversion from camp meals, the park includes a restaurant with the best view around; the restaurant is also adjacent to the swimming pool.

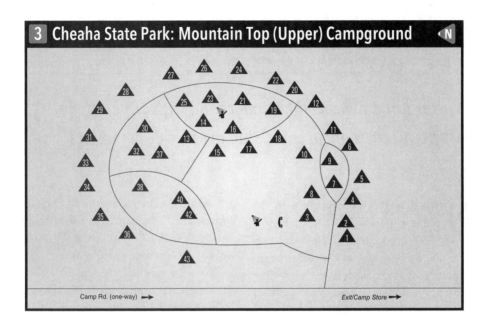

3 Cheaha State Park: Mountain Top (Upper) Campground

Camp Rd. (one-way) ➡

Exit/Camp Store ➡

:: Getting There

From Lineville head north on AL 49 14.2 miles. Turn left onto AL 281. Travel 3 miles. The park entrance is on the right.

GPS COORDINATES N33° 29.172'   W85° 48.794'

4

Coleman Lake Recreation Area

"A beautiful and peaceful campground with large, shady sweet gum trees and a sprinkling of lakeside campsites"

Nestled between mountains in the northern portion of the Talladega National Forest, Coleman Lake Recreation Area offers a beautiful and peaceful campground with large, shady sweet gum trees and a sprinkling of lakeside campsites that make it another great US Forest Service campground.

Coleman is located just outside the town of Heflin. If you're looking at a map, you'll see that the Talladega National Forest splits into two large units totaling more than 380,000 acres. To the west of the state is the Oakmulgee Division, where you will find the Payne Lake Recreation Area (see page 37). To the east is the main Talladega National Forest, which is further subdivided into two smaller districts. In the south there is the Talladega District, where you'll find Cheaha State Park (see page 18) and Lake Chinnabee (see page 28), and to the north is the Shoal Creek District, where the Coleman Lake Recreation Area is located.

:: Ratings

> **BEAUTY:** ★ ★ ★ ★
> **PRIVACY:** ★ ★ ★ ★
> **SPACIOUSNESS:** ★ ★ ★ ★
> **QUIET:** ★ ★ ★ ★
> **SECURITY:** ★ ★ ★
> **CLEANLINESS:** ★ ★ ★

Although fairly close to Atlanta and Birmingham, Coleman feels a world away from big-city hustle and bustle. This is an area to simply come out and unwind.

As with most of the state's US Forest Service recreation areas, Coleman is anchored by a lake, this one covering 21 acres. Nonmotorized or trolling motor-powered boats are permitted, and there are plenty of sloughs and inlets to explore by paddle. Plus, there's fishing for largemouth bass, crappie, bluegill, and catfish. An Alabama freshwater-fishing license is required.

The campground offers prime viewing for wildlife and birds. It's not uncommon for white-tailed deer, as well as foxes, squirrels, and raccoons, to meander through a campsite. That's why you must make sure to pack away food at night. Bird-watchers will be treated to red crossbills with their distinct "jeep-jeep-jeep" calls and the rare red-cockaded woodpecker, named for the color of its plume. You are most likely to spot it in the early morning or just before dusk. Look for the birds in the tops of the tall pine trees.

The famous Pinhoti Trail runs through the recreation area. Pinhoti is an American Indian word meaning "turkey home," another bird often spotted in the area. The US Forest Service and a group of volunteers with the Youth Conservation Corps began trail construction in the early 1970s. Since then, the

ADDRESS: Forest Route 500, Piedmont, AL 36272

OPERATED BY: US Forest Service

CONTACT: 256-463-2272; tinyurl.com/lakecoleman

OPEN: March 15–December 1

SITES: 39

SITE AMENITIES: Gravel pad, fire ring with grate, water, power

ASSIGNMENT: First-come, first-serve

REGISTRATION: Self pay at kiosk

FACILITIES: Flush toilets, showers, playground, lake swimming, fishing

PARKING: At each site

FEE: $12

ELEVATION: 1,142'

RESTRICTIONS:

■ **Pets:** On leash only

■ **Fires:** In fire ring only; use only deadfall

■ **Alcohol:** Prohibited

■ **Vehicles:** 2/site

■ **Other:** Quiet hours 10 p.m.–6 a.m.

---

trail has expanded to more than 130 miles in Alabama, from near the town of Sylacauga to the Georgia state line. From there, the Georgia trail section meanders over mountaintops until it connects to the Appalachian Trail. While you're in camp, keep an eye out for Pinhoti through-hikers. You'll enjoy meeting them and hearing their stories.

The campground contains two unnamed loops. Sites 1–16 are in loop A, and sites 17–39 are in loop B. All have crushed gravel tent pads, a fire ring, water, and power. Between the two loops, you'll find a very nice handicap-accessible bathhouse with hot showers and flush toilets.

You'll find the best sites lakeside in loop B with some nice views of the water, but these are hard to come by since there are only a few.

The Lake Coleman campground does not have a locking access gate, but the US Forest Service rangers do patrol it regularly. The campground is closed in the winter.

Occasionally the forest service performs what is called a prescribed burn, a controlled fire to remove duff building on the forest floor and to stimulate forest growth. Naturally, the campground will be closed during those times. You can check on planned burns at the US Forest Service website at **fs.usda .gov/alabama.**

Then, of course, there are unscheduled wildfires. Please make sure that all fires have been completely extinguished before leaving camp. Fire risk increases during the hot, dry summer or other times when humidity is extremely low.

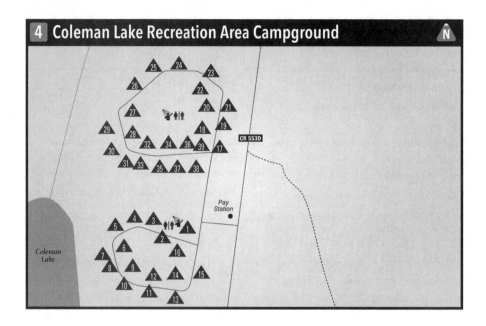

:: Getting There

At the intersection of AL 4 and US 78 in Heflin, turn right onto US 78 East and travel 7.8 miles. Turn left onto County Road 61 and drive 4.3 miles, and turn right onto CR 548. Travel 4.6 miles and bear left onto Forest Route 500. The entrance is on the right in 0.1 mile.

GPS COORDINATES N33° 47.392' W85° 33.378'

5

Deerlick Creek Campground

"Peace and tranquility are the norm at Deerlick Creek Campground."

The **Black Warrior River** has played an important role in Alabama for thousands of years. The river was the lifeblood of American Indians who lived in this area as far back as 1000 A.D. It provided drinking water, fishing, and irrigation for farming, and it also served as a major trade route connecting villages.

The river became an important trade route for Europeans as well after they settled in this region in 1540 and began moving goods and personnel. The waterway eventually flows into the Tombigbee River and ends at the Gulf of Mexico in Mobile.

To this day, the river holds the same importance for these very same reasons. It provides drinking water to the city of Birmingham, and it is a shipping route to the Gulf of Mexico. With the construction of a lock and dam by the US Army Corps of Engineers in 1966, another important role was added to the river's résumé—miles and miles of recreational opportunities, including those found along the banks of Holt Lake.

Holt is a 3,200-acre lake that stretches some 18 miles from end to end, providing

:: Ratings

BEAUTY: ★ ★ ★ ★ ★
PRIVACY: ★ ★ ★ ★
SPACIOUSNESS: ★ ★ ★ ★
QUIET: ★ ★ ★ ★
SECURITY: ★ ★ ★ ★
CLEANLINESS: ★ ★ ★ ★

amazing fishing and boating opportunities—and of course camping.

I can't say enough about the campgrounds operated by the US Army Corps of Engineers. Each provides a wonderful mix of beautiful landscapes and equally beautiful facilities. And one of the best is Deerlick Creek Campground.

It's tucked away in a towering hardwood forest. Here you'll be sleeping under beech trees, oaks, and pines, mainly loblolly; however, the loblolly pines may not be around for long. A nonnative species, loblollies are prone to disease and not resilient to storms. Slowly, many state agencies and nonprofit organizations are removing the loblolly pines and reforesting the area with the native, and much hardier, longleaf.

Peace and tranquility are the norm at Deerlick Creek Campground. You'll find plenty of space between campsites, so you're guaranteed a good amount of privacy, plus it is very quiet.

Hikers will find several short trails, including one on the lake's western bank and another leading to a swimming beach. A road biking trail also provides recreation. And if you like to fish, anglers can choose from four piers.

The campground offers 46 sites altogether, and guests won't find limits on the number of tents that can be pitched per pad, unlike most facilities.

:: Key Information

ADDRESS: 12421 Deerlick Rd., Tuscaloosa, AL 35406	**FEE:** Tent-only site with water and power, $14; site with water and power, $18; waterfront site with water and power, $20
OPERATED BY: US Army Corps of Engineers	
CONTACT: 205-759-1591; reservations 877-444-6777; tinyurl.com/deerlickcreek	**ELEVATION:** 456'
OPEN: March–November	**RESTRICTIONS:**
SITES: 46	■ **Pets:** On 6-foot leash only; not allowed on beach
SITE AMENITIES: Picnic table, fire ring with grill, lantern post, water, power	■ **Fires:** In fire ring or grill only
ASSIGNMENT: By reservation	■ **Alcohol:** Prohibited
REGISTRATION: At gatehouse or by reservation	■ **Vehicles:** 2/site
FACILITIES: Flush toilets, hot showers, laundry, playground, lake swimming, beach, fishing piers	■ **Other:** Quiet hours 10 p.m.–6 a.m.; 2-night minimum stay; reservations can be made 6 months in advance but no later than 2 days prior to arrival; gate locked 10 p.m.–7 a.m.; 2 tents (8 people)/site; 14-day stay limit
PARKING: At each site	

Sites 1–40 offer power, water, a picnic table, a lantern post, a fire ring, and a grill. The tent pads are compact crushed gravel.

If you like to camp with a view, check out sites 5–9, 13–18, and 34–39. All are located high enough above the lake to take it all in. These sites also provide room for two vehicles to park.

But for my favorite spots, seek out the Settler's Camp, sites 41–46. Tent-only sites are normally an afterthought, as operators bank on making their money on RVs, but the primitive sites at Deerlick are phenomenal.

The sites are located just below the campground road on a bluff overlooking a finger of the lake. A short set of wooden stairs leads down to the wide dirt tent pad, picnic table, lantern post, and fire ring with grill. Although called primitive, each site has power. Maybe they should be called semiprimitive? In any case, the view is wonderful and the solitude unbeatable. You'll find a paved parking area just above the sites big enough for two vehicles.

The campground has a spacious and clean central bathhouse with hot showers. A laundry is available here as well. And Deerlick is gated, so there is excellent security. The gate is locked 10 p.m.–7 a.m.

The only downside to spending a night or two at Deerlick Creek Campground is that it's closed November–February—the prime time to view bald eagles in the area.

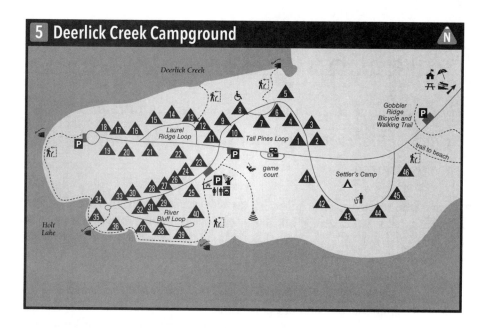

5 Deerlick Creek Campground

:: Getting There

From Tuscaloosa take Lurleen B. Wallace Boulevard North 0.6 mile. Turn right onto Fifth Street/County Road 30. Travel 0.1 mile and turn right, continuing on Fifth Street/CR 30. In 2.4 miles Fifth Street becomes Rice Mine Road. Continue 3.4 miles and turn right onto CR 87/New Watermelon Road. Travel 3.5 miles and turn right onto CR 42/Lake Nicol Road. Travel 3.4 miles and turn right onto CR 89/Deerlick Road. Travel 3.6 miles. The entrance will be on the left.

GPS COORDINATES   N33° 16.295'   W 87° 25.895'

6

Lake Chinnabee Recreation Area

"Those who love to explore nature while camping in a rustic setting will find everything they seek at Lake Chinnabee Recreation Area."

Those who love to explore nature while camping in a rustic setting will find everything they seek at Lake Chinnabee Recreation Area. Located only 6 miles from Cheaha State Park in the Cheaha Wilderness, Lake Chinnabee puts you in closer proximity to nature than the park does, providing easy access to several of the forest's most popular hiking trails.

The recreation area was named for famed Creek chief Chinnabee. He and his tribe adapted and worked with white settlers, ultimately becoming an important ally of General Andrew Jackson during the Creek Indian War of 1813.

The lake that bears the chief's name is relatively small, about 17 acres. It is dammed on the north side by a picturesque spillway. Cheaha Creek, a beautiful mountain stream to the west, feeds the lake. For the anglers among you, this is a great little fishing hole for largemouth bass (an Alabama freshwater-fishing license is required), as well as a great

:: Ratings

BEAUTY: ★ ★ ★ ★
PRIVACY: ★ ★ ★
SPACIOUSNESS: ★ ★ ★
QUIET: ★ ★ ★
SECURITY: ★ ★
CLEANLINESS: ★ ★ ★

paddling lake with plenty of interesting geology, plant life, and sloughs to explore. You can cast your line from the grassy bank near the campground or put in your nonmotorized boat.

The area is also a prime location to explore the wonders of the Talladega National Forest. Several hiking trails ranging from easy to difficult converge at this spot, providing access to even more trails that you can connect to make loops. The forest's most popular hike is the Chinnabee Silent Trail. The *silent* part of the name pays homage to a group of Boy Scouts at the Talladega Institute for the Deaf and Blind who helped build the trail.

The Chinnabee Silent Trail begins near the Cheaha Creek inlet at the western end of Lake Chinnabee and travels along the creek's banks. The creek is rather slow moving in this section, but about 0.5 mile farther the water begins to churn as it cascades down several rock ledges. Here you'll find an amazing natural swimming hole; on hot summer days cool down with a dip in the ice-cold mountain water.

As you hike farther along the climb gets steeper, and you soon find yourself scaling a rock wall on wooden platforms and wooden and stone stairs. Take a look over the railing at a marvelous site—the cascading waters of Devil's Den!

:: Key Information

ADDRESS: Lake Chinnabee Rd., Delta, AL 36258	**PARKING:** At each site
OPERATED BY: US Forest Service	**FEE:** $8
CONTACT: 256-362-2909; tinyurl.com/chinnabee	**ELEVATION:** 760'
OPEN: March–December 1	**RESTRICTIONS:**
SITES: 8	■ **Pets:** On leash only
SITE AMENITIES: Gravel pads, picnic table, fire ring with grate	■ **Fires:** In fire ring only; use only deadfall
ASSIGNMENT: First-come, first-serve	■ **Alcohol:** Prohibited
REGISTRATION: Self pay at kiosk	■ **Vehicles:** 2/site
FACILITIES: Vault toilets, creek swimming, fishing	■ **Other:** Quiet hours 10 p.m.–6 a.m.

At about the 4-mile mark, a small climb leads to the Cheaha Falls Shelter, a building used by backpackers to escape the elements, and just below that is another spectacular three-tier waterfall. All in all, the hike from the lake to the shelter and back is 8 miles round-trip. If you turn around at Devil's Den, it's approximately 4 miles total round-trip.

Other hikes include the Skyway Loop Trail, a steep climb up the side of a mountain from the lake, with nice seasonal mountain streams on top and a nice view. If you are not into mountain climbing, try the much easier Lake Chinnabee Loop Trail circling the lake.

Keep in mind that the Lake Chinnabee Recreation Area is located in the Cheaha Wilderness and is a primitive campground, so unless you want to travel to the towns of Delta, Ashland, or Lineville, all of which are a good 15–30 miles away, make sure that you pack everything you may need. It's about 6 miles to the Cheaha State Park country store, which has limited supplies.

The campsites are relatively close together, so you lose a bit of privacy. Beautiful hardwood trees shade each site. All sites have gravel tent pads, fire rings with grate, and picnic tables. The best campsite is the first one as you enter the campground. The site has a nice view of the lake and surrounding hills, not to mention spectacular views of the fall foliage. The only facilities here are vault toilets.

While the campground isn't gated, US Forest Service rangers regularly patrol it. This can be a busy recreation area. In the spring visitors flock here to see wildflowers, in the summer they come in droves to swim in the stream, and in the fall they come to see the foliage. The Talladega 500 NASCAR race also brings people to the campground to avoid pricey hotels.

Also, the road to the area is narrow, long, and winding, so use caution as you drive down to it. And remember that the campground is closed December–March because the road ices over.

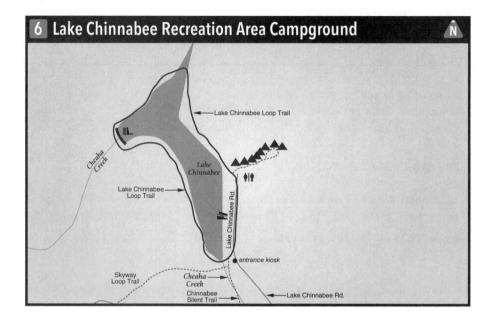

:: Getting There

From Delta travel on AL 9 North 2 miles. Turn left onto Good Hope Delta Road and drive 5 miles. Turn right onto AL 49 North and drive 3.7 miles. Turn left onto AL 281 South (you will pass Cheaha State Park on the right). Travel 4.9 miles. Turn right onto Cheaha Road and drive 3.6 miles. Turn left onto Chinnabee Road and drive 1.1 miles. The entrance is at the end of the road.

GPS COORDINATES   N33° 27.624'   W85° 52.489'

7

Moundville Archaeological Park

"One of the largest American Indian settlements in the country"

This park lets you mix camping with history at an active archeological site. Located just east of Tuscaloosa, Moundville Archaeological Park covers more than 320 acres and features 26 ancient mounds, the remnants of one of the largest American Indian settlements in the country.

The area was inhabited between 1000 and 1450 A.D. during an age known as the Mississippian period. During this time, Moundville was a major political, social, and religious center. Built high atop a bluff on the banks of the Black Warrior River, the settlement can be best described as a planned community. It centered on a tall, plazalike mound that was surrounded by other public buildings, much like a courthouse square.

The mounds are astonishing, with the tallest reaching 55 feet. All have flat tops and were built by piling up baskets full of dirt dug up by hand. The ponds and lakes around the area show where the dirt was originally mined. These mounds were either used as residential homes, as ceremonial sites, or for burials. In the strict social structure of the Mississippian people, the noblemen always had the tallest mound.

The University of Alabama has been excavating this site and bringing the rich history of Moundville to the public since 1869. Over the years researchers have amassed an incredible wealth of knowledge and artifacts about ancient life here, making Moundville a fascinating and beautiful place to explore.

The mounds tower above the grounds and are quite evident as you drive into the park. You can climb to the top of the highest, which offers exceptional views of the wide Black Warrior River far below, or take in the history with a stroll along the Edward T. Douglass Nature Trail. The park's ring road provides excellent biking to the mounds as well.

The museum recently underwent a $5 million renovation and is well worth the visit. Visitors see the Moundville tribes' distinctive pottery, native attire, and vivid displays of life in the settlement. Plus, a 3-D presentation featuring an American Indian medicine maker adds some dazzle.

Camping here is a pleasure, with 31 improved and 5 primitive campsites. In the improved area, sites 3–6 are RV only, but tent campers can use the remaining spots. The sites are very level with no defining

:: Ratings

BEAUTY: ★ ★ ★ ★
PRIVACY: ★ ★ ★ ★
SPACIOUSNESS: ★ ★ ★
QUIET: ★ ★ ★ ★ ★
SECURITY: ★ ★ ★ ★ ★
CLEANLINESS: ★ ★ ★ ★

:: Key Information

ADDRESS: 13075 Moundville Archaeological Park, Moundville, AL 35474

OPERATED BY: University of Alabama

CONTACT: 205-371-2572; moundville.ua.edu

OPEN: March–November

SITES: 29 improved, 5 primitive

SITE AMENITIES: Improved–picnic table, fire ring with grill, water, power; Primitive–picnic table, fire ring

ASSIGNMENT: First-come, first-serve

REGISTRATION: Pay attendant at office

FACILITIES: Flush toilets, hot showers, museum

PARKING: At each site; however, for primitive camping, park only at site 12

FEE: Improved, $12 (senior citizens age 55 and older, $10); primitive, $8; must also pay a one-day park admission: adults, $8; senior citizens, $7; children, $6

ELEVATION: 154'

RESTRICTIONS:

- **Pets:** On leash only
- **Fires:** In fire ring only
- **Alcohol:** Prohibited
- **Vehicles:** 2/site
- **Other:** Quiet hours 10 p.m.-7 a.m.; 2 tents/site; 14-day stay limit

separation except the site marker itself. There isn't a tent pad; instead each site is a grass area. You'll find ample parking for two vehicles and can pitch up to two tents per site.

The primitive sites are located behind site 12. Each has a picnic table and fire ring. Camping is not allowed in site 12 itself, as that is where primitive campers park and access water.

The one central bathhouse is clean, offers hot showers, and more than adequately accommodates the number of campers. Security is outstanding: the gate is locked each night at 9 p.m., and campers receive a code to enter and exit.

The best sites for waking up to an unobstructed view of the mounds are 7 and 9, although you can see the mounds pretty clearly from all but the primitive sites. The best time to visit is in October during the annual Moundville Festival, a weekend-long living history exhibit with demonstrations of native dance, crafts, and community life. Expect crowds, as the festival is often promoted as one of the top 20 in the state. During a visit, I had to park what seemed like a good mile or two from the festivities. With that in mind remember that the park does not take reservations. It's first-come, first-serve, so arrive early. And also keep in mind that the park is closed December–February.

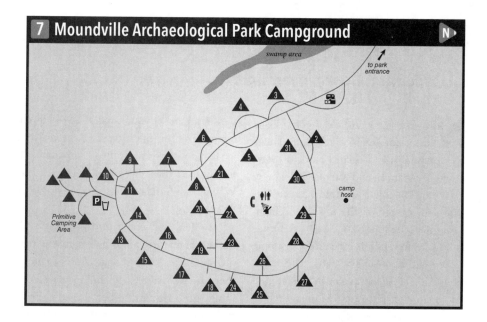

:: Getting There

From Tuscaloosa at the intersection of I-365, I-20, and AL 69, take AL 69 South and travel 13.2 miles. The park entrance will be on the right.

GPS COORDINATES   N33° 00.107'   W87° 38.225'

8

Oak Mountain State Park

"It's a giant outdoor playground."

What do you want to do today? Fish? Swim? Mountain bike? Golf? Hike? Oak Mountain is a giant outdoor playground. You name it and you can find it here.

One of the top three state parks in Alabama and located in the town of Pelham just south of the state's largest city, Birmingham, Oak Mountain is a beautiful example of the southern Appalachians. The hardwoods come alive with color in the fall; the park has numerous water features, such as lakes, streams, and waterfalls; and there's an inspiring lush, green glade in the spring.

Park activities are too numerous to mention in this short profile. Of course there are hiking trails, 51 miles of them actually. One standout is the Blue Trail, named for its blue paint blazes, which eventually leads to breathtaking mountaintop views. The rather strenuous Green Trail climbs straight up a ridge to the top of the spectacular 60-foot Peavine Falls. And the White Trail leads to Maggie's Glen, a beautiful pastoral forest glade with a stream running through it.

For those who would rather ride than walk, you can mountain bike more than 22 miles of trail, bike the park on 7 miles of wide park road, or try your hand at BMX bicycle racing. For the traditionalists among you, what about horseback riding? You can rent a mount from the park and take a guided tour Wednesday–Sunday (guests must be at least 8 years old).

Golfers will enjoy the fact that Oak Mountain features an 18-hole course with a pro shop and driving range. And of course there are park staples, including lake swimming and boat rentals, but also something a bit different—a petting and exhibit farm.

One of Oak Mountain's biggest attractions is the Alabama Wildlife Rehabilitation Center. Each year the center receives almost 1,800 birds, more than 100 species in all, which need medical treatment and rehabilitative care. The birds, as well as other animals, can be viewed both in the center and along the Treetop Nature Trail, where you will see birds of prey that unfortunately cannot be released back into the wild.

Tent camping is unique at Oak Mountain. Overall, every site is perfect, neatly tucked into the forest on hillsides. Many sites have half-height, three-sided cement walls around the tent pad; this was done so that the sites could be leveled and support the berm behind the pad. Each site has a fire ring with grate for grilling and water sources nearby.

Sites 1–3 and 70–72 have the advantage of being near the campground entrance, where there is a small camp store. You'll find a good stock of supplies that you might have left behind there. Sites 47–49 and 64–68 are

:: Ratings

BEAUTY: ★ ★ ★ ★
PRIVACY: ★ ★ ★ ★
SPACIOUSNESS: ★ ★ ★ ★
QUIET: ★ ★ ★ ★
SECURITY: ★ ★ ★ ★ ★
CLEANLINESS: ★ ★ ★ ★ ★

:: Key Information

ADDRESS: 200 Terrace Dr., Pelham, AL 35124

OPERATED BY: Alabama State Parks

CONTACT: 205-620-2527; alapark.com /oakmountain

OPEN: Year-round

SITES: 64 tent sites

SITE AMENITIES: Fire ring, water in the area, picnic tables

ASSIGNMENT: First-come, first-serve

REGISTRATION: Pay attendant at camp store or by reservation

FACILITIES: Flush toilets, hot showers, laundry, playground, lake swimming, fishing, camp store

PARKING: At each site

FEE: Primitive (for 4 people), $16; add $3 for each additional person

ELEVATION: 606'

RESTRICTIONS:

■ **Pets:** On 6-foot leash only; not allowed in buildings or beach area

■ **Fires:** In fire ring only; use only deadfall or purchase wood on-site

■ **Alcohol:** Prohibited

■ **Vehicles:** 1/site

■ **Other:** Quiet hours 10 p.m.–6 a.m.; 1 tent (8 people)/site

located by one of the campground's four bathhouses, which are modern with hot showers and very clean. The best sites for a view of the lake are sites 42B and 64–66.

You can register for a campsite at the campground's front gate until 9 p.m., but because the park is in such close proximity to the state's largest city, it is packed most

any time. To guarantee a spot, call ahead to make reservations (call Monday–Friday, 9 a.m.–4 p.m.).

Security is excellent at Oak Mountain. Park enforcement rangers patrol the campgrounds 24 hours a day and man the locked gate so that registered campers can come and go after-hours.

8 Oak Mountain State Park Campground

:: Getting There

From Birmingham take I-65 South about 14 miles. Take Exit 246 and turn right onto AL 119. Travel 80 yards and take the first left onto Oak Mountain Park Road. Travel 1.5 miles and turn left at the four-way stop onto John Findley Drive, where you will see the park entrance straight ahead. Travel 5.9 miles (John Findley Drive will turn into Oak Mountain Park Road again), and turn left onto Campground Road. The campground is 0.3 mile ahead.

GPS COORDINATES   N33° 20.994'   W86° 43.230'

9

Payne Lake Recreation Area

"If you're looking for solitude, then you'll find it at Payne Lake Recreation Area."

Solitude. **If that's what** you're looking for, then you'll find it at Payne Lake Recreation Area in the heart of the Oakmulgee Unit of the Talladega National Forest. Don't be confused. There are two Talladega National Forests on most maps: one to the east side of the state, where Alabama's tallest mountain, Cheaha, is located, and this one to the west.

The Oakmulgee Unit was declared a national forest on January 21, 1935, and encompasses more than 150,000 acres of upland pine forest. The woodland is one of the last remnants of a much larger ecosystem that at one time stretched from Texas to the Carolinas. The forest you see looks virtually the same as it did when Europeans first arrived in the area in the 1500s.

The remote location makes this the perfect home for many species of birds, including hawks, wrens, nuthatches, turkeys, yellow-billed cuckoos, and the rare red-cockaded woodpecker. You can view these and many more along one of the recreation area's two interpretive hikes—the Payne Lake Nature Trail, which also includes a nice trip down to the lakeshore, or the Eastern Nature Trail, which stretches from the southern end of the lake past the East Side Campground and ends at the north tip of the 110-acre lake.

As with many of Alabama's national forests, the Oakmulgee is experiencing a rebirth. At one time, 90 million acres of longleaf forest covered the Southeast, but today only a fraction of this native species of pine remains. The current dominant species, loblolly, is prone to disease and cannot stand up to the punishment Mother Nature often brings to the area with hurricanes and tornados.

The U.S. Department of Agriculture, along with many public and private organizations and volunteers, are working to restore longleaf pines throughout Alabama, including here in the Oakmulgee, and the rangers there will be happy to talk to you about the effort. Work has been completed in both the East Side and West Side Campgrounds and both are open for business.

With that being said, let's get down to camping. As mentioned earlier there are two camp loops, the West Side and East Side. The West Side loop consists of 18 sites. Sites 1–3 and 6–9 are improved with water and electricity. Sites 4–5 and 10–18 have water only. Sites 1–10 are prime locations, offering a splendid view of the lake to wake up to. Sites 4 and 5 are on the uphill side, so you

:: Ratings

BEAUTY: ★ ★ ★ ★ ★
PRIVACY: ★ ★ ★ ★
SPACIOUSNESS: ★ ★ ★
QUIET: ★ ★ ★ ★
SECURITY: ★ ★ ★
CLEANLINESS: ★ ★ ★ ★

:: Key Information

ADDRESS: 9901 AL 5, Brent, AL 35034	**FACILITIES:** Flush toilets, hot showers, laundry, playground, fishing
OPERATED BY: US Forest Service	**PARKING:** At each site
CONTACT: 205-926-9765; tinyurl.com /paynelake	**FEE:** West Side, $16; East Side, $10
OPEN: West Side–year-round; East Side–October 1–Memorial Day	**ELEVATION:** 265'
SITES: 56	**RESTRICTIONS:**
SITE AMENITIES: Gravel pad, fire ring, grill, picnic table, lantern post, water, power	■ **Pets:** On leash only
ASSIGNMENT: First-come, first-serve	■ **Fires:** In fire ring only
	■ **Alcohol:** Prohibited
REGISTRATION: Pay attendant at office or at honor box	■ **Vehicles:** 2/site
	■ **Other:** Quiet hours 10 p.m.–6 a.m.

still have a nice view even with other campers in the lower sites. The bathhouse has nice hot showers, is heated for wintertime visits, and is very clean; it's just the right size for the number of sites and visitors to the recreation area.

The East Side Campground is more secluded and set back from the lake. These sites, 19–55, each have a picnic table, fire ring, and basic dirt pad. The East Side Campground is seasonal, open October 1–Memorial Day. The bathhouse on this side of the lake is closed, so you will have to walk or drive to the West Side bathhouse.

The East Side Campground benefits from its location on the park's Eastern Nature Trail and near the beach. Speaking of which, while the lake is a great swim, remember that there are no lifeguards, so you swim at your own risk.

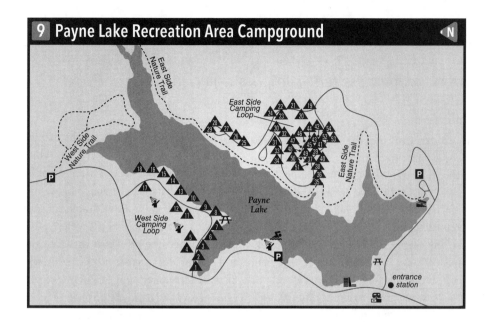

9 Payne Lake Recreation Area Campground

:: Getting There

From Moundville take AL 69 South 8.9 miles. Turn left onto County Road 29. Travel 9.1 miles. Turn left onto CR 25 North. Travel 2.4 miles and make a slight left onto CR 71. Travel 1.1 miles. The entrance will be on the right.

GPS COORDINATES   N32° 52.836'   W87° 26.820'

10

Pine Glen Campground

"A true wilderness tent-camping experience"

If you're looking for a true wilderness tent-camping experience, then look no further than the Pine Glen Recreation Area, ideally located for great hiking and fishing adventures deep in the forest and far from the crowds of the popular Cheaha State Park.

Pine Glen lies within the Shoal Creek Ranger District of the Talladega National Forest. President Franklin Roosevelt established the forest in 1936, combining two units under the umbrella of the name Talladega: the Oakmulgee on the west side of the state and Talladega to the east.

In 1945 the Talladega Unit was further divided into two districts, the Talladega (where you will find the state's highest mountain, Cheaha) and Shoal Creek Ranger Districts. By the way, the name Talladega is a Creek Indian word meaning "border town."

At the time the Talladega Unit was subdivided, 30% of the land was clear-cut, cultivated, and vacated farmland. Today, the 380,000 acres offer a wilderness wonderland teeming with wildlife, wildflowers, birds, creeks, streams, lakes, and waterfalls. Being away from the crowds in a peaceful mountain valley and next to the Choccolocco

:: Ratings

> **BEAUTY:** ★ ★ ★ ★
> **PRIVACY:** ★ ★ ★
> **SPACIOUSNESS:** ★ ★ ★ ★
> **QUIET:** ★ ★ ★ ★
> **SECURITY:** ★ ★
> **CLEANLINESS:** ★ ★ ★

Wildlife Management Area means that you are bound to see plenty of wildlife. White-tailed deer, bobcats, squirrels, and gopher tortoises are not uncommon.

The area is also a bird-watcher's paradise with hundreds of bird species calling the hardwoods home. These include wood and mallard ducks, green-winged teals, warblers, wild turkeys, and rare red-cockaded woodpeckers, to name only a few.

Many people do not realize that the mountains of the Talladega National Forest are actually part of the Appalachian Mountain range, which ends, or begins depending on your orientation, just south of here near Birmingham.

Like the Coleman Lake Recreation Area, Pine Glen has a world-famous attraction running through it—the Pinhoti Trail, a long-distance hiking route that currently begins near the town of Sylacauga and winds its way through the Talladega Mountains some 130 miles to the Georgia state line. At that point backpackers can continue along the Georgia Pinhoti Trail until it connects to the Appalachian Trail. You'd be surprised to know that many hikers actually begin their trip in Key West, Florida, and end it in Canada, some 5,500 miles away from their starting point—and they use the Pinhoti Trail to get there. Many of these hikers stop over in Pine Glen. Be sure to talk with them about their adventure.

If you're into hiking yourself, this stretch of the Pinhoti is a nice walk in the

:: Key Information

ADDRESS: Forest Route 500, Heflin, AL 36264

OPERATED BY: US Forest Service

CONTACT: 256-463-2272; tinyurl.com/pineglencamp

OPEN: Year-round

SITES: 23

SITE AMENITIES: Picnic table, fire ring with grate

ASSIGNMENT: First-come, first-serve

REGISTRATION: Self pay at kiosk

FACILITIES: Vault toilets, fishing

PARKING: At each site

FEE: $3

ELEVATION: 1,022'

RESTRICTIONS:

■ **Pets:** On leash only

■ **Fires:** In fire ring only; use only deadfall

■ **Alcohol:** Prohibited

■ **Vehicles:** 2/site

■ **Other:** Quiet hours 10 p.m.–6 a.m.

woods. It is a short 3-mile hike to Sweet-water Lake, a very pretty mountain reservoir formed by a small flood-control dam. Along the route you will be treated to beautiful tulip poplar trees that have yellow blooms in late spring. If you're a determined hiker, you can walk the 6 miles to the Coleman Lake Recreation Area from here. Just remember that it's 6 miles one way. You have to come back.

I've heard good things about the fishing in Shoal Creek, which runs along the north side of the campground. Redeye black bass and redear sunfish are the catches here, and as always, an Alabama freshwater-fishing license is required.

The Pine Glen Recreation Area is located just to the west of the town of Heflin, where the Shoal Creek Ranger District's headquarters is located. But the ride to town from the campground is a bumpy and winding trip down dirt forest roads. Be cautious:

It's easy for oncoming vehicles to make wide turns around the sharp curves.

For a primitive campground the sites are very nice. Each campsite has level grass areas on which to pitch your tent, with hardwoods and pines providing plenty of shade. A fire ring and picnic table is located at each site, and a community water spigot is available at the campground entrance.

Little to no foliage between campsites reduces your privacy a bit, but ample spacing between the sites makes up for that. For a little more solitude I suggest choosing a campsite on the west side of the campground because it appears that most people stay closer to the entrance gate. And while no site is directly on Shoal Creek, the sites along the camp road to the north as you enter the campground offer the best view.

While the campground lacks a security gate, the area is patrolled by US Forest Service rangers.

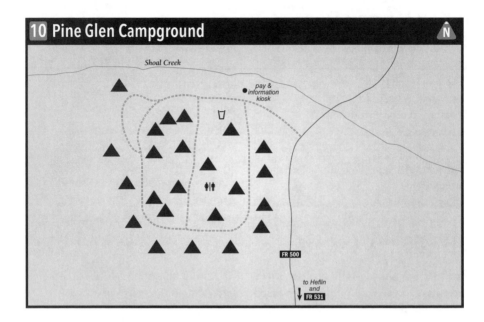

:: Getting There

At the intersection of AL 46 and US 78 in Heflin, turn right onto US 78 East and travel 0.3 mile. Turn left onto Old Edwardsville Road. Cross railroad tracks and immediately turn right onto Oxford Street. Travel 2.4 miles. Turn left onto Forest Route 548, a dirt road, and travel 1.9 miles. Come to a Y-intersection and take the left fork onto FR 531. Travel 2 miles. Turn right onto FR 500, and travel 0.5 mile. The campground is on the left.

GPS COORDINATES N33° 43.484'   W85° 36.096'

11

Tannehill Ironworks Historical State Park

"The hand-built stone furnace towers over the grounds and is a marvel to see."

High atop a pedestal on a ridge overlooking the city of Birmingham is a statue of Vulcan, the Roman god of metalworking. It was erected in honor of the region's rich iron-producing history, and much of that history can be traced to one of the earliest iron forges in the area at Tannehill Ironworks Historic State Park.

It all began in 1830 when Pennsylvanian Daniel Hillman came to the area and built a forge along the banks of the raging waters of Roupes Creek. Well before he had a chance to see the fortune that the furnace would bring, Hillman passed away, and a local farmer, Ninian Tannehill, purchased it.

Tannehill used slave labor to hand-cut sandstone bricks, which were used to construct three tall furnaces. By 1862 the furnaces were in full operation, producing 20 tons of iron a day, the bulk of the output being used for cannons and artillery for the Confederate Army.

:: Ratings

> **BEAUTY:** ★ ★ ★ ★
> **PRIVACY:** ★ ★ ★
> **SPACIOUSNESS:** ★ ★ ★
> **QUIET:** ★ ★ ★ ★
> **SECURITY:** ★ ★ ★ ★
> **CLEANLINESS:** ★ ★ ★ ★

Needless to say the furnace became a prime target of the Union Army. Destroying the furnace would virtually disarm the Confederacy. In March 1865 General James Wilson rode in with the Eighth Iowa Cavalry and shelled and set fire to the foundry; the event would later become known as Wilson's Raid on Alabama. At the same time, the Union torched the cabins of the slaves who built and worked the furnace, killing 600 during the attack.

After the war a businessman purchased the ironworks, but resurrecting its past glory proved impossible due to hard economic times, and the site was abandoned to be reclaimed by nature.

The ironworks remained dormant and hidden under the overgrowth for a century until the state of Alabama, along with several colleges, resurrected the furnace. Over several years archeological digs uncovered the old blower house and the main furnace itself, which was rebuilt and fired up once again in 1976.

The furnace and surrounding area were eventually made into a historic state park, Tannehill, which encompasses more than 1,500 acres of hardwood forest just north of Bessemer and has been added to the National Register of Historic Sites. Over the years several attractions, including a demonstration village, have been added. Everything from basket-making to quilting

:: Key Information

ADDRESS: 12632 Confederate Pkwy., McCalla, AL 35111	**PARKING:** At each site
OPERATED BY: Alabama Historic Commission	**FEE:** Improved (for 4 people), $21; primitive (for 4 people), $16; add $4 for each additional person
CONTACT: 205-477-5711; tannehill.org	**ELEVATION:** 511'
OPEN: Year-round	
SITES: 176 improved, 100 primitive	**RESTRICTIONS:**
SITE AMENITIES: Improved—picnic table, fire ring with grill, water, power; Primitive—fire ring, most have picnic tables	■ **Pets:** On leash only
	■ **Fires:** In fire ring only
ASSIGNMENT: First-come, first-serve	■ **Alcohol:** Prohibited
REGISTRATION: Pay attendant at camp store	■ **Vehicles:** 2/site
FACILITIES: Flush toilets, hot showers, playground, camp store, museum	■ **Other:** Quiet hours 10 p.m.–6 a.m.; 1 tent (4 people)/site; registration 7 a.m.–10 p.m.; 14-day stay limit

to pottery and, of course, blacksmithing, is displayed here to show visitors what life was like in the mid–19th century.

The park has several excellent hiking trails, totaling about 5 miles, that will take you along the banks of the beautiful blue-green waters of Roupes Creek, down stagecoach roads, and to the slave cemetery.

The park's Iron and Steel Museum of Alabama offers a fascinating journey that harks back to the years the foundry rivaled any in the Northeast.

And of course, the centerpiece of the park is the main furnace and blower. The hand-built stone structures tower over the grounds and are a marvel to see.

For camping you have quite a selection; 176 improved sites and 100 primitive sites are divided into three separate loops. Improved sites have the comforts of home: water, electricity, a picnic table, a grill, and a fire ring. Primitive sites have fire rings, and most also have picnic tables.

While many campsites seem to be close together, they still offer considerable privacy. Campground 1 has 42 sites (101–142) and is mostly used by RVs. Campground 2 has 22 sites (200–221) that are ideal for tent campers. The bathhouse for both loops is located just outside of Campground 1 on the west side. Campground 2 is also located close to the old-time country store, which has a good selection of camping necessities. Sites 200–210 in this loop are particularly nice. They are located right on the banks of Mud Creek (also known as Roupes Creek). The creek is wide and usually has a good flow. After a good winter or spring rain, the blue-green waters roar past your campsite.

Campground 3 has 112 sites (301–409) and its own bathhouse. It is a little removed from the country store and park attractions, but it is much quieter than the other two campgrounds, which are in the thick of things. The loop is also along the banks of Mud Creek, with sites 331–335 sitting right next to the creek itself.

The primitive loop is the farthest removed from the main park attractions. It

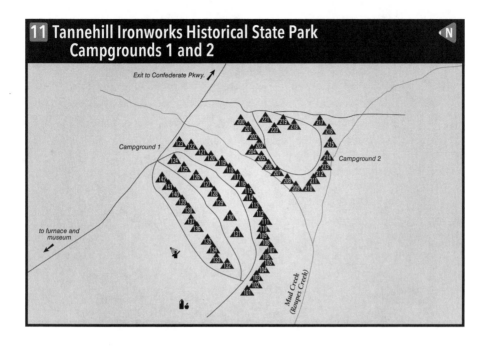

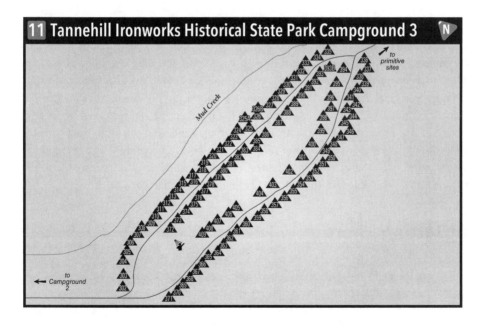

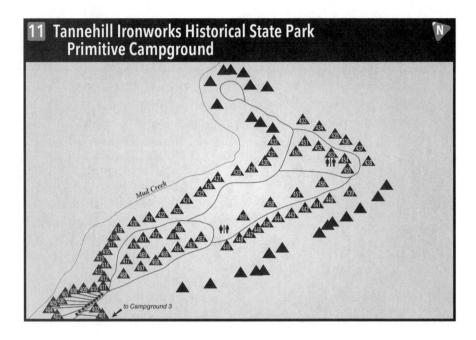

11 Tannehill Ironworks Historical State Park Primitive Campground

has 100 sites altogether. What I found here were 52 marked sites and many unmarked sites scattered around the loop. Two vault toilets are the only facilities here. As with the improved campgrounds, the primitive loop is located on the banks of Mud Creek. For the best views of the creek (and to be lulled to sleep by the rushing waters), try for sites 400–432. As I said, there are a number of unmarked sites here, with only fire rings scattered about the loop. The sites you may want to avoid here are those unmarked sites to the east (right) of sites 438–449. They are located at the bottom of a hill, and I imagine that runoff during a rain could make for a miserable weekend.

All sites are level with grass and dirt pads. You'll find two clean, heated bathhouses, one just outside of Campground 1 and one inside Campground 3. The bathhouses are large, capable of handling the huge crowds that come for Trade Days (held the third weekend of the month March–November) and for the mammoth Halloween celebration at the campground. And when I say huge crowds, I mean *huge*. Sites come at a premium during Trade Days and are on a first-come, first-serve basis, so get there early.

:: Getting There

From McCalla take I-20 West/I-59 South 7.9 miles. Take Exit 100 and turn left onto AL 216. Travel 0.2 mile. AL 216 becomes Bucksville Road. Continue another 0.4 mile and make a slight left onto Tannehill Parkway. Travel 2.7 miles. Tannehill Parkway becomes Confederate Parkway. Continue 0.1 mile. The entrance is on the left.

GPS COORDINATES   N33° 15.129'   W87° 04.189'

Mountain Region

12

Buck's Pocket State Park

"One of the state's best-kept secrets"

Tucked away in the sandstone pocket of a canyon in northeast Alabama, you'll find 2,000-acre Buck's Pocket State Park. It's described by many as one of the state's best-kept secrets with beautiful landscapes and excellent hiking and fishing.

The park is located within a canyon rimmed by sandstone walls more than 400 feet tall. More on that in a moment, but first, what about that name?

Legend has it that the name came from the American Indians who lived in the region thousands of years ago and used the canyon's rocky overhangs for protection from the elements. As the story goes, a hunter tracked a large buck to the edge of a canyon ledge. Confronted by the hunter and with no place else to go, the buck jumped into the pocket.

Buck's Pocket State Park Campground is situated along the banks of a tributary of Lake Guntersville called South Sauty Creek. Large boulders line its banks, and when it gets full, the creek puts on a spectacular blue-green water show as it races to Morgan's Cove and the lake.

:: Ratings

BEAUTY: ★ ★ ★ ★
PRIVACY: ★ ★ ★
SPACIOUSNESS: ★ ★ ★
QUIET: ★ ★ ★ ★
SECURITY: ★ ★
CLEANLINESS: ★ ★ ★ ★

As you enter the park, the sign at the office reads A HAVEN FOR DEFEATED POLITICIANS. As another story goes, some prominent elected officials, including governors, came to Buck's Pocket to lick their wounds after suffering defeat at the ballot box.

One of the highlights of a visit here is a high outcrop called Point Rock. It towers some 400 feet above the base of the campground, offering spectacular views of the surrounding bluffs that form the canyon. At the top you'll likely run into rock climbers practicing on the steep bluff. The top also offers a beautiful picnic area.

You can either drive or hike to the top and those views. If you choose the latter, be warned: the hike is a steep 3.5-mile out-and-back from the campground with a hefty elevation gain.

If you like fishing, then head down the camp road to secluded Morgan's Cove, which has a boat launch, pier, and huge bass. A state freshwater-fishing license is required. Even if you don't like to fish, the visit is well worth it, especially on cool mornings with a light fog—a beautiful sight.

As for overnighting, the improved campsites are excellent but limited. Tent pads are level with light compact gravel. Each site has water, power, a picnic table, and a fire ring with grill.

The best sites are 1–17, which are located very close to the banks of South Sauty Creek. The creek's rushing water will lull you to sleep.

:: Key Information

ADDRESS: 393 County Road 174, Grove Oak, AL 35975

OPERATED BY: Alabama State Parks

CONTACT: 256-659-2000; alapark.com /buckspocket

OPEN: Year-round

SITES: 19 improved, 11 primitive

SITE AMENITIES: Improved—picnic table, fire ring with grill, water, power; Primitive—picnic table, fire ring

ASSIGNMENT: First-come, first-serve

REGISTRATION: Pay attendant at office or after-hours honor box at entrance

FACILITIES: Flush toilets, hot showers, playground, boat launch, fishing pier

PARKING: At each site

FEE: Improved with water and power, $21; improved with water, power, and sewer, $22; primitive, $15; add $4 for additional tent

ELEVATION: 678'

RESTRICTIONS:

■ **Pets:** On leash only

■ **Fires:** In fire ring only

■ **Alcohol:** Permitted

■ **Vehicles:** 2/site

■ **Other:** Quiet hours 10 p.m.–6 a.m.

While the improved campsites are nice, the primitive sites leave something to be desired. They are located on the south side of the park at the base of Point Rock in a small run, which could get pretty wet in a good rain. Several sites also sit on an incline, making pitching a level tent difficult. There are a few picnic tables, but they look as though they are moved from site to site by campers. The bottom line: To enjoy camping at Buck's Pocket, spend the extra money for the improved sites.

This is not a gated park, so in that sense, security is lacking. If you arrive after-hours, pay at the honor box; otherwise, pay at the office located at the park's entrance. The bathhouses are adequate with flush toilets and hot showers, but they are showing their age.

Peak visitation comes during spring when the creek is full, as well as during fall when visitors seek the autumn colors and crisp mountain air. If you plan on going during these times, make sure to get there early to get a spot.

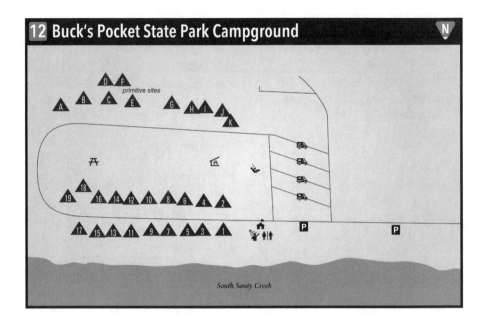

:: Getting There

From Guntersville take AL 227 South 17.2 miles. Turn left onto County Road 50. Travel 1.8 mile. Turn left onto CR 20. In 0.6 mile CR 20 becomes CR 19. Continue north on CR 19 1.2 miles. CR 19 turns to the right, take the slight left onto CR 557. Travel 0.5 mile and turn left onto CR 173. The entrance to the park is on the right in 0.5 mile.

GPS COORDINATES   N34° 28.531'   W86° 02.938'

13

Cane Creek Canyon Nature Preserve

"Amazing geology, breathtaking waterfalls, crystal-clear springs and streams, and wildflowers await you."

Amazing **geology,** breathtaking waterfalls, crystal-clear springs and streams, and hundreds of varieties of wildflowers all await on the 400 acres known as the Cane Creek Canyon Nature Preserve. Oh, and by the way, you can camp there, too.

The preserve is owned by Jim and Faye Lacefield. In 1976 they purchased a small parcel of land at what is now the south end of the preserve and built a home. What lay to the north was an amazing and beautiful landscape that they felt needed to be protected. In 2000 the couple purchased the land from a timber company and set to work building a labyrinth of hiking trails. The result is one of the most beautiful locations in Alabama.

Along the many trails, visitors will see towering rock walls and shelters. These walls tell the geologic history of the region dating to ancient times, when the area was part of a barrier island off of what is known as Pangaea, a large landmass comprised of all of today's current continents joined together.

:: Ratings

BEAUTY: ★ ★ ★ ★ ★
PRIVACY: ★ ★ ★ ★ ★
SPACIOUSNESS: ★ ★ ★ ★ ★
QUIET: ★ ★ ★ ★ ★
SECURITY: ★ ★ ★
CLEANLINESS: ★ ★ ★ ★ ★

Eventually the continents drifted apart and this area was lifted up out of the ocean.

Time and the elements have since carved this canyon, forming astounding rock formations that American Indians used for shelter thousands of years ago during the Mississippian era. Throughout the preserve you will come across these shelters, many sporting cascading waterfalls.

In spring Cane Creek comes alive with vibrant colors bursting forth from wildflowers in the glades dotting the property. In the winter, you can really see the geologic features of the canyon with a bird's-eye view from atop the Point, a small peak about 300 feet above the canyon floor.

Cane Creek Canyon Nature Preserve is simply a wonderland with way too much to describe here, but let me tell you: Jim and Faye Lacefield are the most gracious hosts you'll ever find, willing to impart their knowledge of the canyon and point out things you may miss. While I was there, Jim was justly proud in showing me a rare swamp metalmark butterfly. It's no wonder that the Nature Conservancy, which partners with the Friends of Cane Creek, rate the preserve as one of the most public-friendly preserves anywhere.

Five designated primitive camping areas are within the preserve—Small Point, the Point, Linden Meadows, Creekside, and Devil's Hollow. All with the exception

:: Key Information

ADDRESS: 201 Loop Rd., Tuscumbia, AL 35674

OPERATED BY: Privately owned—Jim and Faye Lacefield

CONTACT: 256-381-6301; tinyurl.com/canecreekcanyon

OPEN: Year-round

SITES: 5

SITE AMENITIES: Dirt pad, stone fire ring, picnic table; Linden Meadows also has a picnic shelter

ASSIGNMENT: First-come, first-serve

REGISTRATION: Download permit from tinyurl.com/canecreekcanyon (a Facebook page) or contact the Friends of Cane Creek Canyon Nature Preserve at 256-381-6301

FACILITIES: Portable toilets

PARKING: Only at Small Point campsite; remaining sites are backcountry. If not camping at Small Point, park in the designated parking next to the Lacefields' house.

FEE: Free

ELEVATION: 747'

RESTRICTIONS:

■ **Pets:** On leash

■ **Fires:** By daily request (check with the owners first) and only as conditions allow; in fire ring only; use only deadfall

■ **Alcohol:** Prohibited

■ **Vehicles:** 1/Small Point; no vehicles allowed elsewhere

■ **Other:** Quiet hours 10 p.m.–6 a.m.; reservations (a completed permit) must be received at least 24 hours in advance; group size limited to 6, except Small Point, which can accommodate 16; camp in designated sites only; campers must arrive before 4 p.m.; no entering or leaving after dark; 2-night stay limit

of Small Point require that you park at the Lacefields' house and hike in to the campsite. The closest is Small Point, about 0.3 mile from the parking area. Next is the Point at about 0.5 mile away, followed by Linden Meadows at 0.75 mile, Creekside at 1.5 miles, and finally, the farthest out, Devil's Hollow, at 2.5 miles. Remember, you'll be hiking into a canyon, and what goes down must come up, so be very conscientious about how much gear you bring along.

The one exception to backcountry camping is Small Point. You are allowed to drive one vehicle to the site. Each campsite has modern and clean privies, a stone fire ring, and a picnic table. Linden Meadows also has a picnic shelter. Please check with the Lacefields before building a campfire to make sure that no fire advisory is in effect, and only use deadfall. As for security, the front gate is locked after-hours, and you will not be permitted to leave or enter the campground after dark.

The five sites all have their own unique character. Linden Meadows is named for the fragrant linden trees in the area. The site is located next to the beautiful, clear Cane Creek. The Point is so named because of its location on a peak. Creekside, well, I think you know where that name came from. The campsite is located near an area known as Old Beaver Pond. These long-extinct beaver ponds have created beautiful glades graced with wildflowers that bloom spring–fall. The most interesting of all the sites is Devil's Hollow, which is near a huge rock shelter with seasonal waterfalls nearby.

While camping at Cane Creek Canyon Preserve is free, you must reserve your spot no later than 24 hours in advance. Visit

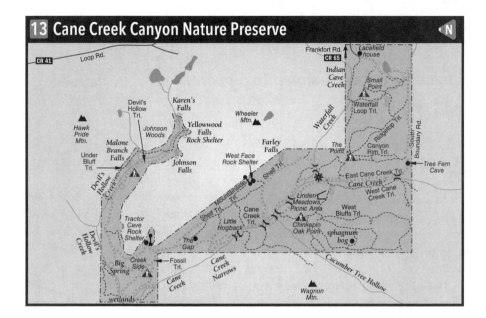

13 Cane Creek Canyon Nature Preserve

the Friends of Cane Creek on Facebook to download a reservation permit or contact Faye Lacefield at the number listed in the Key Information to have one sent to you.

Pitch camp and explore the canyon at your leisure, but please be sure to follow Leave No Trace practices and ethics to protect the canyon for generations to come.

:: Getting There

From the intersection of US 72 and Frankfort Road/County Road 65 in Tuscumbia, take Frankfort Road/CR 65 South 7.5 miles. Turn right onto Loop Road. Travel 0.1 mile and bear left onto the dirt road (a small CANE CREEK CONSERVANCY sign leads the way). Travel 0.5 mile to the preserve's entrance. Parking is clearly marked and to the left.

GPS COORDINATES   N34° 37.350'   W87° 47.668'

14

Cathedral Caverns State Park

"A magnificent excursion into Alabama's underground wonders"

Alabama has more than 4,100 known caves, two of which have been transformed into state parks. The first is Rickwood Caverns (see page 90); the second is yet another magnificent excursion into Alabama's underground wonders, Cathedral Caverns.

This subterranean complex was formed in limestone as waters from an ancient ocean percolated down through the ground, carving out these massive caves. Originally called Bats Cave, the property was first opened for public tours in the 1950s by Jacob Gurley. He renamed the cave Cathedral Caverns after his wife reportedly said that the soaring ceilings in many of the chambers with towering stalagmites reminded her of a cathedral.

The property was declared a National Natural Landmark in 1972. The state bought the 461-acre property in 1987, but it wasn't opened as a state park until 2000. In addition, Alabama's Forever Wild, a program that purchases property of historical or environmental significance, bought additional property adjacent to the park in 2008 to further the cave's protection.

It has been said that the cave is more beautiful than better-known caves such as Mammoth in Kentucky or Luray in Virginia. The only difference is that Cathedral is a well-kept secret, but one that is becoming more and more known each year.

The cave boasts of many world records, including having the largest opening of any commercially operated cave, measuring 126 feet wide and 25 feet tall. It's also home to the world's largest stalagmites, Goliath, which measures 45 feet tall and 243 feet in circumference.

In addition, the cave holds the world record for the largest stalagmite forest, the largest flowstone wall, the largest frozen waterfall, and a record that the state describes as "the most improbable stone formation in the world," a stalagmite that stands 35 feet tall but is only 3 inches wide.

Two things strike people when they first enter the cave. First is the sheer enormity of the entrance. Stand along the overview high above the cave entrance and you'll see that people walking down the cement pathway to start their tour are dwarfed by the gaping expanse.

The other is the fresh air within the cave. Caves are normally dank and musty, but Cathedral has its own filtration system, the Mystery River, which runs the length of the cavern and continually circulates fresh

:: Ratings

BEAUTY: ★ ★ ★ ★
PRIVACY: ★ ★ ★ ★
SPACIOUSNESS: ★ ★ ★ ★
QUIET: ★ ★ ★
SECURITY: ★
CLEANLINESS: ★ ★

:: Key Information

ADDRESS: 637 Cave Rd., Woodville, AL 35776

OPERATED BY: Alabama State Parks

CONTACT: 256-728-8193; alapark.com/cathedralcaverns

OPEN: Year-round

SITES: 13

SITE AMENITIES: Fire pit

ASSIGNMENT: First-come, first-serve

REGISTRATION: At park store

FACILITIES: Portable toilets, community water spigot, picnic area

PARKING: At each site

FEE: $13

ELEVATION: 642'

RESTRICTIONS:

■ **Pets:** On leash

■ **Fires:** In fire pit only; use only deadfall or purchase at office

■ **Alcohol:** Prohibited

■ **Vehicles:** Multiple allowed

■ **Other:** Quiet hours 10 p.m.–6 a.m.

oxygen throughout its passages. The river may run just a few inches deep or reach more than 30 feet during flooding.

A cave tour covers about 1.3 miles and takes around 90 minutes. The tour is wheelchair accessible and runs every two hours September–March, and every hour April–August. The tour does not operate on January 1, Thanksgiving Day, or December 25.

The gift shop offers a wide selection of cave memorabilia, T-shirts, and information on the cave. The staff loves to talk about caves, spelunking, and the park itself. While you are there, children and even adults may want to try panning in the park's Gem Flume. Pick up a $6 bag of mining dirt at the gift shop.

The campsite is strictly primitive and has a few drawbacks, but the Department of Conservation and Natural Resources, which oversees the Alabama State Park system, plans to develop an improved campground in the future.

The existing site is about 0.5 mile from the gift shop and cave entrance. Heading down Cathedral Caverns Road, you will make a left turn onto Cave Road. Almost immediately you will see a dirt road fork to the right, which leads to the campsites. When you arrive, however, continue straight down Cave Road approximately 0.5 mile to the gift shop, where you will register.

Facilities are very limited, so bring all of the groceries you need for your stay. There is a men's and women's portable toilet located at the entrance of the campsite area. A few sites, 7 and 10–15, have fire rings.

The best sites are in the back corner of the campground, specifically sites 8–12, which provide plenty of shade and are far enough away from the road that car noise will not be an issue. Sites 1, 2, 14, and 15 are more out in the open with little shade, but they are spacious. Sites 2–7 are parallel to Cathedral Caverns Road; although the road has light traffic, the noise and the location could be bothersome to some.

The park manager lives across the street from the campground, so in case of emergency you can either contact the gift shop, if open, or the park manager.

:: Getting There

From Scottsboro take US 72 West 14.2 miles. Turn left onto County Road 63. Travel 8.2 miles. Turn left onto Cathedral Caverns Road. Travel 0.1 mile to the park entrance.

GPS COORDINATES   N34° 34.322'   W86° 13.703'

15

Clear Creek Recreation Area

"A great place to pitch your tent and explore the wonders of the Bankhead National Forest"

Northwest Alabama has a 190,000-acre treasure called the William B. Bankhead National Forest. Within its boundaries you will find more diversity both geologically and biologically than in any other national forest in the state. Clear Creek Campground offers a great place to pitch your tent to explore these wonders.

Located on the banks of Lewis Smith Lake, Clear Creek is touted as one of the most popular national forest recreation areas in the state, and it's no wonder. The Bankhead has something for everyone. To the north is the famous Sipsey Wilderness, known as the Land of a Thousand Waterfalls. (Just remember that many waterfalls in Alabama run seasonally.) A short drive from the campground leads to Natural Bridge, the longest such natural rock formation east of the Mississippi. And the forest is blanketed with seemingly endless trails—more than 150 miles of biking and mountain biking trails, almost 100 miles of hiking trails, and hundreds more miles

:: Ratings

BEAUTY: ★ ★ ★ ★
PRIVACY: ★ ★ ★ ★
SPACIOUSNESS: ★ ★ ★ ★
QUIET: ★ ★ ★ ★
SECURITY: ★ ★ ★ ★ ★
CLEANLINESS: ★ ★ ★ ★ ★

of equestrian trails. The forest's rivers also welcome canoeing and kayaking.

But you don't have to leave base camp for a great weekend. Clear Creek Campground itself has a 1.5-mile mountain biking trail plus a 2.5-mile hiking trail called the Raven Interpretive Trail, which highlights the region's amazing flora. In addition, Clear Creek has lake swimming, basketball and volleyball courts, horseshoe pits, and playgrounds. And just outside the gate, you'll find the Pine Torch Church Historic Site. This nondenominational church was built circa 1850 with poplar logs, and it reportedly gained its name from the pine torches that were used to light the church at night. The church is still in use today, holding services at 10 a.m. every Sunday.

You'll also find exceptional fishing here, with Kentucky and hybrid striped bass being the main catches.

Clear Creek has 102 campsites in four loops—Fox Loop with sites 1–34, Hoot Owl with sites 35–60, Fawn Loop with sites 61–83, and Bear Loop with sites 84–105. All have gravel pads, water, power, a picnic table, and a barbecue grill. They are either first-come, first-serve or can be reserved by phone, with the exception of those in Bear Loop, which are by reservation only.

Every Clear Creek site appeals with ample spacing between each unit and plenty of shade from the native hardwoods. You

:: Key Information

ADDRESS: 8079 Fall City Rd., Jasper, AL 35503

OPERATED BY: US Forest Service

CONTACT: 205-384-4792; reservations 877-444-6777; tinyurl.com/clearcreekrecarea

OPEN: Mid-March–mid-November

SITES: 102

SITE AMENITIES: Gravel pads, picnic table, fire ring, grill, lantern post, water, power

ASSIGNMENT: First-come, first-serve or by reservation (Bear Loop reservation only)

REGISTRATION: At entrance station; after-hours: 205-384-4792

FACILITIES: Flush toilets, showers, playground, boat ramp, lake swimming, fishing, basketball and volleyball court, horseshoe pit, ice machine, firewood

PARKING: At each site

FEE: Single site, $19; single waterfront site, $20; double site, $38; double waterfront site, $40

ELEVATION: 770'

RESTRICTIONS:

■ **Pets:** On leash only; not allowed in swimming area

■ **Fires:** In grill only

■ **Alcohol:** Prohibited

■ **Vehicles:** 2/site; additional can park in overflow parking area for $4/day

■ **Other:** Quiet hours 10 p.m.–6 a.m.; 6 people/site

will find, though, that Fox Loop has a bit more canopy and shade than the other loops and Hoot Owl Loop has better spacing and offers more trees between sites.

The absolute best sites are 1, 3D, 4D, 5, 24D, and 26D in Fox Loop and 35–39, 57, 59, and 60 in Hoot Owl Loop which are right on the water. You'll pay a little extra to camp at these sites, $1 for a single site or $2 for a double, but don't scrimp now! That little bit is well worth it to pitch your tent along the beautiful blue-green lake.

You can find campground hosts in three of the loops—Fox Loop at site 34, Fawn Loop at site 73, and Bear Loop at site 90. The hosts are great people and will go out of their way to help you anyway they can.

Each loop has its own bathhouse, with an extra one between the Fox and Hoot Owl Loops. The medium-size, handicap-accessible facilities are very clean with single hot showers. The gate to the campground is locked at 10 p.m., which provides excellent security. Campers receive a combination to enter after-hours. And those needing to register after-hours can contact the on-duty host at the phone number posted on the kiosk just outside of the entrance station.

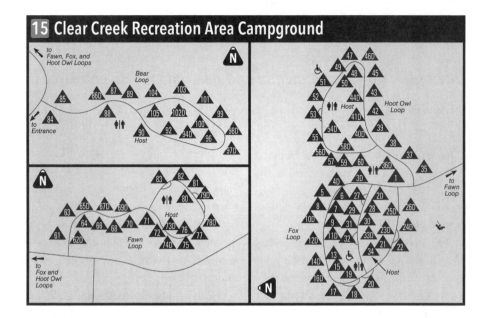

15 Clear Creek Recreation Area Campground

:: Getting There

From the intersection of Old US 78 and AL 195 in Jasper, take AL 195 North 4.1 miles. Turn right onto Fall City Road. Travel 6.7 miles. The campground entrance station is on the left.

GPS COORDINATES   N34° 00.747'   W87° 15.914'

16

Corinth Recreation Area

"One of the most ecologically and geologically diverse areas in the state"

The **William B. Bankhead** National Forest, one of four such forests in the state of Alabama, is perhaps the most ecologically and geologically diverse. It also has an identity crisis.

The forest was established in January 1918 as the Alabama National Forest with only 66,000 acres. In June 1936 it was renamed for the main river that flowed through the region, the Black Warrior. Finally in 1942 it was renamed yet again for William B. Bankhead, an influential Alabama congressman who played important roles in helping establish New Deal legislation with President Franklin Roosevelt. He was also the father of actress Tallulah Bankhead.

Today the forest covers more than 190,000 acres and is home to amazing natural wonders, including old-growth oak, maple, and black gum trees. In fact, along Bee Branch in the nearby Sipsey Wilderness, hikers come to admire a 150-foot-tall poplar tree more than 500 years old.

The thick forest canopy hides deep gorges and canyons and beautiful clear mountain streams and rivers. Waterfalls dot the forest and are always nearby. The most popular locations include Caney Creek Falls, located off County Road 2 near the town of Double Springs, and the falls of the Sipsey Wilderness. The 25,000-acre Sipsey is called Land of a Thousand Waterfalls, and after one visit in the spring, you will understand why.

The Bankhead also has abundant wildflowers. Hundreds of varieties, including white trilliums and lady's slippers, bloom spring–fall. All of this beauty is accessible via the 80 miles of hiking trails (including some that are handicap-accessible) or the 40 miles of equestrian trails; the beauty is also visible by paddlers on the 60-mile Sipsey, a National Wild and Scenic River.

Bankhead includes six recreation areas, including Corinth. Located just outside of the town of Double Springs on the banks of Lewis Smith Lake, Corinth, along with the Clear Creek Recreation Area, is sometimes called Birmingham's backyard because city dwellers flock to the areas in the summer. Still, Corinth remains peaceful, quiet, and beautiful.

Its lake location offers excellent fishing. Wet your line and try your hand at landing Kentucky, largemouth, or striped bass. And of course the swimming in Lewis Smith Lake is great!

In all, Corinth has 60 sites, 52 improved and 8 primitive. The improved sites are in two loops, Yellow Hammer and Firefly, all

:: Ratings

BEAUTY: ★ ★ ★ ★
PRIVACY: ★ ★ ★ ★
SPACIOUSNESS: ★ ★ ★ ★
QUIET: ★ ★ ★ ★
SECURITY: ★ ★ ★ ★ ★
CLEANLINESS: ★ ★ ★ ★ ★

:: Key Information

ADDRESS: 2540 County Road 57, Double Springs, AL 35553

OPERATED BY: US Forest Service

CONTACT: 205-489-3165; reservations 877-444-6777; tinyurl.com/corinthrec

OPEN: Mid-March–mid-November

SITES: 52 improved, 8 primitive

SITE AMENITIES: Improved–gravel pads, picnic table, grill, lantern post, water, power; Primitive–dirt pad, picnic table, fire ring, grill, community water spigots

ASSIGNMENT: First-come, first-serve or by reservation

REGISTRATION: At entrance station or by reservation

FACILITIES: Flush toilets, hot showers, boat ramp, lake swimming, fishing, play field, ice machine, firewood

PARKING: At each site

FEE: Improved, $22; primitive, $15

ELEVATION: 770'

RESTRICTIONS:

■ **Pets:** On leash only; not allowed in swimming area

■ **Fires:** In grill only

■ **Alcohol:** Prohibited

■ **Vehicles:** 2/site; additional can park in overflow parking area for $4/day

■ **Other:** Quiet hours 10 p.m.–6 a.m.; 6 people/site

with gravel pads, power, water, a lantern post, a picnic table, a grill, and a fire ring, and the dispersal-type primitive area has tables, simple dirt pads, and fire rings. The primitive area also provides several community water spigots. All sites have a thin canopy covering them, enough to provide shade to help beat the heat.

Ample space separates every site, so you won't lack for privacy. The best sites, of course, are along the lake. Those would be Yellow Hammer sites 15, 16, and 18 and Firefly sites 38–41.

The campground provides three clean and recently remodeled bathhouses, two in the Yellow Hammer Loop and the third in

Firefly. Each roomy unit has a separate men's, women's, and unisex facilities, all handicap-accessible, and have a single hot shower. The men's side includes a baby-changing station.

The campground gate is locked at night, and campers are provided with a security code for access. If you arrive late, call the number posted on the kiosk outside of the entrance station for after-hour registration.

Once again you will find the volunteer camp hosts extremely friendly and knowledgeable. They work the entrance station during the day and help clean up around the campground. Hosts can be found in the Yellow Hammer Loop at site 1 and in Firefly at site 30.

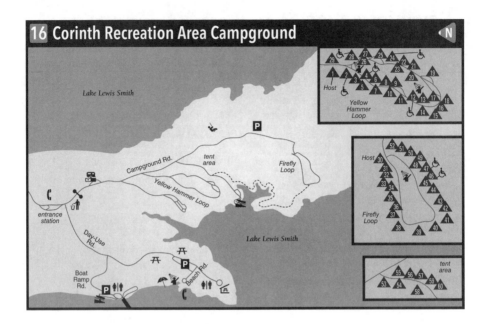

:: Getting There

From the intersection of County Road 53/Snoddy Road and AL 74/US 278 East in Double Springs, take AL 74/US 278 East 3.6 miles. Turn right onto CR 57 and travel 2.8 miles. Turn right into the Corinth Recreation Area. The entrance station is about 0.4 mile straight ahead.

GPS COORDINATES N34° 06.542' W87° 19.290'

17

DeSoto State Park

"Spend a weekend or more exploring waterfalls, deep canyons, and wildflowers at the Home of Mother Nature."

High atop Lookout Mountain, above Fort Payne, stands another gem of the Alabama State Park system: DeSoto State Park. Nicknamed "The Home of Mother Nature," DeSoto is one of those perfect parks where you can pitch camp and spend a weekend or more exploring waterfalls, deep canyons, wildflowers, and much more and still not experience everything it has to offer.

DeSoto State Park encompasses more than 3,500 acres, which includes a portion of Little River Canyon. Known as the Grand Canyon of the East, the gorge, formed by its namesake river, is the deepest canyon east of the Mississippi. The portion of the canyon within the park boundaries is along the West Fork of Little River. The view of the raging water below is breathtaking from high atop the rim at the lodge and along the park's DeSoto Scout Trail. Remember, however, water flow is seasonal, so during times of drought the river may be very shallow.

The park abounds with waterfalls and more than 20 miles of hiking trails leading to them. Among the falls you can venture to are

Laurel, Indian, Lodge, Azalea Cascade, and Lost Falls. The best time for viewing waterfalls is winter, early spring, and late fall.

Don't miss DeSoto Falls. Located 6 miles from the park along the main fork of Little River, it plummets 104 feet into a gorge.

In addition to the plethora of hiking trails, visitors also find 11 miles of mountain biking paths and a 2.5-mile family bike loop.

Aside from waterfalls, DeSoto's other big draws are wildflowers and fall foliage. Blooms of every imaginable color and species, including pink lady's slippers, mountain laurels, and dwarf irises, to name a few, emerge in early spring and peak in mid-May. The park hosts a Wildflower Saturday the first Saturday of May. Throughout the day guided tours take visitors to see the kaleidoscope of colors.

Later in the year, the hardwoods of Lookout Mountain begin to change color and put on a spectacular show themselves. As park rangers are quick to tell you, *historically* colors peak mid-October–mid-November. Like the weekend of Wildflower Saturday in May, this time of year is very busy, so it's best to make reservations well in advance.

While you're here, don't miss the park's Friday- and Saturday-evening nature programs. A ranger or volunteer covers far-ranging topics—such as wildflowers, raptors, reptiles, geology, and more—at the park's large campfire ring between the improved and primitive campgrounds.

:: Ratings

BEAUTY: ★ ★ ★ ★ ★
PRIVACY: ★ ★ ★
SPACIOUSNESS: ★ ★ ★ ★
QUIET: ★ ★ ★ ★
SECURITY: ★ ★ ★ ★ ★
CLEANLINESS: ★ ★ ★ ★

:: Key Information

ADDRESS: 7104 DeSoto Pkwy. NE, Fort Payne, AL 35967

OPERATED BY: Alabama State Parks

CONTACT: 256-845-5075; alapark.com/desotoresort

OPEN: Year-round

SITES: 94 improved, 20 primitive

SITE AMENITIES: Improved—picnic table, grill, water, power; Primitive—fire ring

ASSIGNMENT: First-come, first-serve or by reservation

REGISTRATION: Pay at country store or by reservation

FACILITIES: Vault toilets, hot showers, community water spigot, laundry, pool, fishing, country store

PARKING: Improved—at site; Primitive—along designated parking spaces on the campground road

FEE: Improved (March–October, Sunday–Thursday, and November–February, daily), $28.50; improved (March–October, Friday–Saturday), $31.30; primitive, $13; add $5.35 for additional tent

ELEVATION: 1,471'

RESTRICTIONS:

■ **Pets:** On leash only

■ **Fires:** In fire ring only; use only dead-fall or purchase at office

■ **Alcohol:** Prohibited

■ **Vehicles:** 2/site

■ **Other:** Quiet hours 10 p.m.–6 a.m.; 8 people/site; late arrivals visit DeSoto State Park Lodge or pitch a temporary camp behind the country store; cancellations must be made 72 hours in advance; make holiday weekend reservations 3 months in advance

Other park activities include geocaching, fishing, and swimming. A nature center covers the area's wildlife.

The camping is amazing at DeSoto. The park's improved and primitive sites both have excellent security. The improved area has a gate with keypad; the primitive has a bar gate with pad lock. Campers receive the combination or key upon registration. Remember to return the key in the drop box at the country store when leaving.

The improved campground has all the amenities you would expect, including compact crushed-gravel pads, water, electricity, and fire rings. The sites are a bit close together, so you lose a little privacy, but all in all the sites are surprisingly nice and quiet considering the proximity. The two bathhouses, or comfort stations as the park describes them, are brand-new and modern with hot showers. They're even heated for winter visitors. (The park, by the way, is absolutely gorgeous in snow.)

The country store is amply stocked with items you might have forgotten, such as firewood, drinks, snacks, and, of course, souvenirs.

Primitive sites have grass or dirt pads. There are vault toilets here as well as a community water spigot across from sites 10 and 11. The Quarry Trail and Silver Blaze hiking trail pass this loop, providing easy access to Lost Falls.

One interesting—and convenient—feature for tent campers is the late-arrival area. Located behind the country store and the nature center, a temporary site has been set up so you can pitch your tent after-hours. Simply register the next morning at the store. You will need to park your vehicle at the store and walk back to the site. A sign points the way.

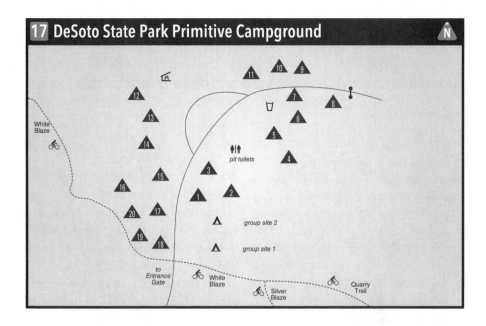

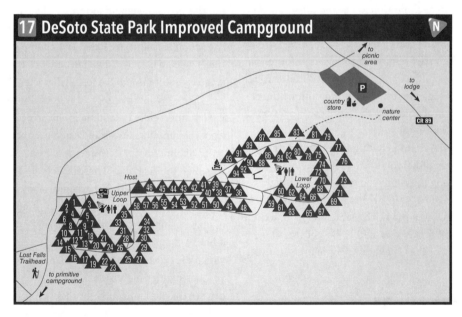

:: Getting There

From Fort Payne take County Road 81 West 7.4 miles. Turn right onto CR 148/ CR 275. Travel 3.7 miles. The camp store is on the left.

GPS COORDINATES   N34° 30.058'   W85° 37.090'

18

Dismals Canyon Conservancy

"You will be treated to some truly amazing landscapes and adventure."

If you haven't guessed by now, the western side of the Mountain Region is dotted with canyons and gorges. Let's add another one to the list: the Dismals Canyon Conservancy. Located in the town of Phil Campbell, the Dismals are privately owned. Within the boundaries of this 85-acre property, you will be treated to some truly amazing landscapes and adventure.

As with similar areas in the region, such as Cane Creek and the Sipsey Wilderness, Dismals Canyon was once part of a vast ancient ocean. This area was believed to have been part of a primeval swamp. More than 300 million years ago it was lifted through geologic forces. Over millenniums, the elements carved out the sandstone to form this beautiful canyon.

A 1.5-mile hiking trail along the canyon floor allows you to view this beauty up close. Along the route you will pass such sights as Weeping Bluff, which resembles an American Indian maiden. Water seeps down the rock face and is said to be her tears for the loss of the Chickasaw people in the canyon.

:: Ratings

BEAUTY: ★ ★ ★ ★ ★
PRIVACY: ★ ★ ★
SPACIOUSNESS: ★ ★ ★
QUIET: ★ ★ ★ ★
SECURITY: ★ ★ ★ ★ ★
CLEANLINESS: ★ ★ ★

Other features include Temple Cave, where Paleo people once used the giant rock overhang for protection; the Grotto, where an earthquake sheared large boulders off the canyon wall, forming natural bridges; and Secret Falls. The source of the falls is an underground stream that pops out of the Earth's surface 0.75 mile upstream from the canyon. Within only 100 feet of the waterfall, 27 species of native trees can be found, including the first state champion tree in Franklin County. A champion tree is the largest of its species in a county or state. The champion tree here is an Eastern Canadian hemlock that stands 138 feet tall and 8.9 feet in diameter.

The canyon has a second waterfall near its entrance called Rainbow Falls, created from the tumbling waters of Dismals Branch.

One final natural wonder is a little critter called the dismalite. These insects are larvae found only in certain parts of the world. They thrive in the canyon's damp, humid climate. Clinging to the rock walls they emit a bluish-green light to attract flying insects, which quickly become dinner. Dismals Canyon has regular nighttime tours, where you can see this magnificent light show for yourself. Tour times change throughout the year, so check with the camp store, and be sure to bring your flashlight. With all of this beauty it's no wonder that the Dismals Canyon has been named a National Natural Landmark.

If you are looking for a little more adventure, Dismals Canyon is located a short drive

:: Key Information

ADDRESS: 901 County Road 8, Phil Campbell, AL 35581

OPERATED BY: Privately owned

CONTACT: 205-993-4559; dismalscanyon.com

OPEN: June–October, daily; March–May and November, Saturday–Sunday; closed December–February

SITES: 18

SITE AMENITIES: Dirt pad, fire ring, grill, trash can

ASSIGNMENT: First-come, first-serve; Sleeping Water or Caveman by reservation only

REGISTRATION: At office

FACILITIES: Flush toilets, hot showers, creek swimming, canoeing, guided tours, camp store

PARKING: At each site; parking for Caveman site is near bathhouse

FEE: Boy Scouts (for 4 people), $43; Caveman (for 4 people), $43; Creek (for 4 people), $27; Dead Water Bluff (for 4 people), $36; Sleeping Water (for 4 people), $48; additional $5 cleanup fee for each site; costs for additional person vary per site; must also pay a one-day park admission: adults, $10; children age 11 and younger, $6; seniors age 60 and older, $9

ELEVATION: 818'

RESTRICTIONS:

■ **Pets:** On leash only; not allowed in swimming area or camp store

■ **Fires:** In fire ring or grill only; obey posted NO FIRE warning signs; use only deadfall

■ **Alcohol:** Prohibited

■ **Vehicles:** 1/site; not allowed at Caveman site

■ **Other:** Quiet hours 11 p.m.–7 a.m.; swimming is at own risk; no hiking, canoeing, or biking after sunset unless accompanied by Dismals guide

away from Bear Creek Canoe Run, a fast and fun ride with several class II+ and III rapids along its 30-mile stretch. You can rent a canoe and hop a shuttle to the put-in at the Dismals camp store. Check with the store for current pricing and schedules.

With all of this natural beauty to protect, it's no wonder that the Dismals Canyon Conservancy has kept camping primitive, allowing only limited tent camping. Visitors can choose from 18 sites, all considered backcountry (you have to walk your gear in). The walk, however, is short. The sites are grouped into six areas: Bath House, Boy Scouts, Creek, Sleeping Water, Dead Water Bluff, and Caveman, and each are distinctive.

The most nondescript sites at the Dismals are the Bath House and Boy Scout campsites. Bath House is, as the name implies, located just a few feet away from the bathhouse. There are two sites here that are basically grass tent pads with a fire ring each. The Boy Scout campsite is located on a hardwood-shaded hilltop a short walk along a trail from the bathhouse. This campsite differs from the others at the Dismals in that it is a group camp area with room for six tents (up to 20 people), a communal fire ring, and a picnic table.

Three of the sites—Creek, Dead Water, and Sleeping Water—are located across AL 8 to the north of the main park entrance. The Creek site is situated along the banks of Dismals Branch, a nice flowing creek that later forms the falls and flows through the bottom of the canyon itself. Dead Water

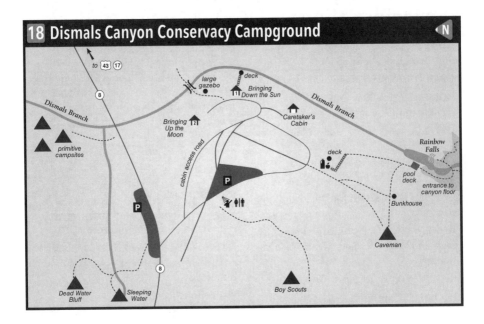

18 Dismals Canyon Conservacy Campground

is a little north of the Sleeping Water site, with easy access to visit a nearby waterfall. Sleeping Water has its own small rock shelter and waterfall (remember that waterfalls are seasonal in Alabama). Needless to say, Sleeping Water is the most popular site at the Dismals.

The second-most popular site is Caveman, which is located at the southern end of the canyon rim near the canyon entrance. This site is highlighted with a 30-foot-tall rock shelter where you can actually pitch a small tent.

The number of people and tents permitted differs for each site. Caveman and Dead Water can take 10 people each and two tents. As noted earlier, Bath House has two sites and each accommodates six people and one tent, while the Boys Scouts site allows six tents for 20 people. Sleeping Water has room for 15 people and three tents. Creek has two sites for two tents and up to 10 people.

The bathhouse is adjacent to the camp store's parking lot. It's clean with plenty of room and two hot showers. In the men's side, be sure to keep the shower curtain closed. The front door tends to open in such a way that you might be putting on a show for anyone outside. Other than that, the bathhouse is very nice.

:: Getting There

From the intersection of County Road 16/College Road and AL 237 in Phil Campbell, take CR 16 3.2 miles. Turn left onto AL 17/US 43 South. Travel 1.1 miles and turn right onto CR 8 and drive 0.7 mile. The large stone entrance to the canyon is on the left.

GPS COORDINATES   N34° 19.642'   W87° 46.950'

19

Elliott Branch Campground

"A beautiful campground on some of the cleanest recreational waters in the South"

In the early 1930s, the Tennessee Valley Authority (TVA) embarked on an enormous task: the creation of a dam system to supply low-cost power to the region, supporting a thriving river system by minimizing flood damage but maintaining maritime navigation, and stimulating economic growth in the region. To do this and do it right the TVA had to purchase more than 1 million acres of land and create 37 reservoirs in five of the seven states in the Tennessee Valley. In the late 1960s, the TVA created four new reservoirs in northwest Alabama that became known as the Bear Creek Water Control Project. Today this project is under the control and management of the Bear Creek Development Authority.

In the resulting years, the authority has created 15 separate public use areas, providing a wide range of recreational opportunities, including fishing, boating, swimming, picnicking, and, of course, camping. One of those campgrounds is Elliott Branch.

Elliott is located on the banks of Little Bear Creek Reservoir, about 13 miles southwest of the town of Russellville. Because

:: Ratings

BEAUTY: ★ ★ ★ ★
PRIVACY: ★ ★ ★ ★
SPACIOUSNESS: ★ ★ ★ ★
QUIET: ★ ★ ★ ★
SECURITY: ★ ★ ★ ★
CLEANLINESS: ★ ★ ★ ★

there is very little residential development on the reservoir, or any of the Bear Creek reservoirs for that matter, the lake is rated as having some of the cleanest recreational water in the South. Many also consider the reservoir, with its towering limestone bluffs, as the prettiest of the Bear Creek lakes.

Paddlers will enjoy floating a portion of the nearby 34-mile Lower Bear Creek Canoe Trail. The trail is a leisurely trip that's great for families. If you had the time, it could take you all the way to the Pickwick Landing Dam in Tennessee.

With its deep channels and brushy bottom, the reservoir is a fishing paradise. The main catches are members of the black bass family—largemouth, smallmouth, and spotted. Crappie, catfish, and bream are also plentiful. You can bank fish, or because Elliott Branch sports a cement boat ramp, you can launch your boat. Be sure to get an Alabama freshwater-fishing license before heading out.

Your first stop upon arriving at Elliott Branch will be at the country store on the right. This is where you'll register and meet the friendly folks manning the store. When I arrived, the staff was just stirring a huge pot of boiled peanuts that gave the store a wonderful aroma. The store isn't fancy but has enough items stocked in case you forgot to bring something along.

In all there are 30 improved sites at Elliott Branch, each with a gravel pad,

:: Key Information

ADDRESS: Elliott Branch Rd., Hodges, AL 35571	**PARKING:** At each site
	FEE: $15
OPERATED BY: Bear Creek Development Authority	**ELEVATION:** 738'
CONTACT: 256-332-4392; 877-367-2232; bearcreeklakes.com	**RESTRICTIONS:**
OPEN: Mid-March–mid-October	■ **Pets:** On leash only; not allowed in beach areas
SITES: 30	■ **Fires:** In grill only
SITE AMENITIES: Gravel pad, picnic table, grill, lantern post, water, power	■ **Alcohol:** Prohibited
ASSIGNMENT: First-come, first-serve	■ **Vehicles:** 2/site
REGISTRATION: At camp store	■ **Other:** Quiet hours 11 p.m.–6 a.m.; 1 tent (8 people)/site; lanterns must be hung on provided posts
FACILITIES: Hot showers, flush toilets, playground, boat ramp, lake swimming, fishing pier, camp store	

power, water, a grill, a picnic table, and a lantern post. All sites have plenty of shade provided by the numerous oak trees, and each has good spacing to assure privacy. With a minimal number of sites, you will find this to be an exceptionally quiet campground.

One bathhouse is located between the two camping loops. The facility is small in size but big enough for the number of campers. The bathhouse is very clean with one hot shower.

For the kids a playground is near the cabins, just down a side road from the camp store, and for the kid in all of us, the swimming here is great. The campground is on a finger of land that juts out into the lake. A small beach, just a few dozen yards away from the camp store and at the south end of a little bay, keeps swimmers away from the main body of water and safe from boat traffic. It is roped off for safety, so you can't go too far into deep water.

Gates are locked at 11 p.m. Campers who need to leave or return after-hours should contact the on-duty ranger. The number will be provided upon registering.

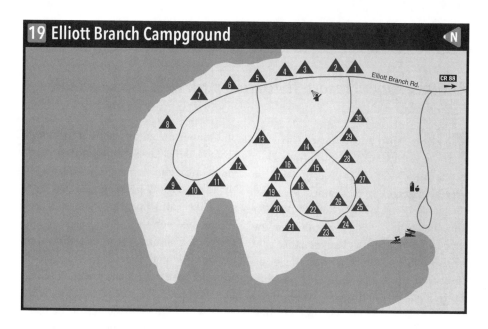

:: Getting There

From Russellville take AL 24 West 13 miles. Turn left onto County Road 88. Travel 2.4 miles and turn left onto Elliott Branch Road. The camp store is 0.1 mile ahead on the right.

GPS COORDINATES   N34° 26.867'   W87° 57.940'

20

Joe Wheeler State Park

"Another superb resort-style state park with many amenities"

The first thing you'll notice when you travel northwest Alabama—from Florence to Muscle Shoals to Decatur—is that everything seems to be named Wheeler: Wheeler National Wildlife Refuge, Wheeler Dam, and Wheeler Highway. All bear the name of Joe Wheeler, a Georgia native who has the unique distinction of serving as an officer for both the Confederate Army during the Civil War and the US Army in the Spanish-American and Philippine-American Wars. His efforts on the battlefield earned him the nickname "Fighting" Joe Wheeler. Between his tours of duty with the military, Wheeler was elected to the U.S. House of Representatives in 1880, where he remained until 1900.

While many streets, buildings, and dams are named after Wheeler, only one beautiful Alabama state park, on the northern banks of his namesake lake, bears his name.

Joe Wheeler is another superb resort state park with many amenities. Visitors find playgrounds, boat rentals, and a gift shop. If you get tired of normal camp fare, then try the park's Daniella's Restaurant, which features excellent breakfast, lunch,

:: Ratings

BEAUTY: ★ ★ ★ ★
PRIVACY: ★ ★ ★ ★ ★
SPACIOUSNESS: ★ ★ ★ ★
QUIET: ★ ★ ★ ★
SECURITY: ★ ★ ★ ★ ★
CLEANLINESS: ★ ★ ★ ★ ★

and dinner menus as well as a memorable seafood buffet on Saturday nights. And if you're into tennis or golf, then head to the park's courts or 18-hole course.

Hikers will find three separate trails, two named for the color blazes marking the path. The first, the Yellow Blaze Trail, a 2.5-mile loop trail, leads to a nice view of Wheeler Lake by the dam. The trailhead can be found near the park's cabin area, across the river on the south side of the dam. The second is the 1.8-mile Blue Blaze Trail that follows the banks of Wheeler Lake where First Creek flows in and through the park's day-use area.

The third path, the 0.5-mile Campground Trail, is just a nice walk in the woods that begins at the end of the primitive camping area and loops around to the banks of the lake.

The park is known as the fishing headquarters for Wheeler and Wilson Lakes. Anglers from around the world come to test the deep waters along the rocky bluffs. Park visitors have two options: one is to bank or boat fish in Wheeler Lake, and the other is fishing in First Creek, a tributary on the north side of the campground. Bass, including smallmouth, white, and hybrid striped, is the name of the game here. On First Creek you can try your hand at largemouth bass, crappie, or catfish. Just remember to have your Alabama freshwater-fishing license at the ready.

Wheeler has a great little swimming area along the lakeshore. The beach is

:: Key Information

ADDRESS: 4403 McLean Dr., Rogersville, AL 35652

OPERATED BY: Alabama State Parks

CONTACT: 256-247-1184; reservations 800-252-7275; alapark.com/joewheeler

OPEN: Year-round

SITES: 116 improved, 30 primitive

SITE AMENITIES: Improved—gravel or dirt pads, picnic table, fire ring, grill, water, power, sewer; Primitive—dirt or grass pads, picnic table, fire ring with grill, community water spigots

ASSIGNMENT: First-come, first-serve or by reservation

REGISTRATION: At campground office or call 256-247-5461 after-hours

FACILITIES: Flush toilets, hot showers, laundry, Wi-Fi, playground, lake swimming, beach, fishing, golf course, tennis courts, camp store

PARKING: At each site

FEE: Improved (for 4 people/November–February), $22; improved (for 4 people/March–October), $25; primitive (for 4 people/November–February), $13; primitive (for 4 people/March–October), $16; add $5 for additional tent

ELEVATION: 598'

RESTRICTIONS:

■ **Pets:** On leash only; not allowed in beach areas or buildings

■ **Fires:** In fire ring or grill only; use only deadfall

■ **Alcohol:** Prohibited

■ **Vehicles:** 2/site

■ **Other:** Quiet hours 10 p.m.–6 a.m.; 1 tent (8 people)/site, extra tent allowed for children; 2-night minimum stay March–October, Saturday–Sunday; 3-night minimum stay on holiday weekends; 14-day stay limit

inviting, the water is cool, and it has a really nice restroom facility with outdoor shower.

One word about the campground—excellent! Each of the 116 improved and 30 primitive sites has plenty of shade and more-than-adequate spacing between units, which means that it is very quiet.

The improved sites are split into three loops: Section A has 42 sites, section B has 48, and section C has 25. As always, the waterfront ones are best. In section A those are sites 24–26; in section B sites 17, 20, 22, 24, and 26–28; and in section C sites 7–10.

Each loop has its own clean bathhouse featuring three hot showers and plenty of space. The facilities, which are handicap-accessible, include an outside sink for washing dirty dishes (but not, FYI, for fish

cleaning). You'll also find a laundry at the check-in station.

Every site has gravel pads, power, water, a picnic table, a grill, and a fire ring. Some sites' power boxes are a little removed from the picnic table or tent pad, so you may want to bring an extension cord.

The sites in the primitive loop feature dirt or grass pads, a picnic table, a fire ring, and a grill. Four community water spigots are arranged around the loop.

Campground security is excellent, with an electronic gate locked every night at 10 p.m. Each camper receives the numeric combination to access the gate after-hours. And one more note: The campground hosts a Sunday chapel service in the section B loop directly across from the loop's bathhouse.

20 Joe Wheeler State Park Campground

:: Getting There

From the intersection of County Road 66/McLean Drive and US 72 in Rogersville, take McLean Drive south 4.4 miles. The campground entrance station is straight ahead.

GPS COORDINATES   N34° 48.448'   W87° 18.789'

21

Lake Guntersville State Park

"A total recreation resort"

When I first visited Lake Guntersville State Park, it was for a little book about hiking that I wrote a decade ago. What a beautiful place. The blue-green waters of its namesake 6,000-acre reservoir shimmered alongside the campgrounds, and it quickly became a favorite. But Mother Nature is always at work, and in the spring of 2011 a massive EF3 tornado barreled through north Alabama, leaving a path of death and destruction in its wake. Lake Guntersville State Park stood in the path of the storm.

I drove up to the park along AL 227 and couldn't believe my eyes. At first I thought that a timber company was clear-cutting, but then it became clear what had happened. The woods on the north side of the park were devastated.

Heading to the campground and talking to the attendants at the camp store, I learned that no one was seriously injured there, but that most of the campgrounds had been rendered unusable. Five bathhouses were destroyed, and several trails had to be closed because of downed trees or the danger of widow makers, trees that have toppled but are hanging precariously

high above the trail and can come down at any moment.

But Alabamians are resilient and Alabama State Parks has been working hard to bring the park back to life, and it has. All 321 sites, as well as the damaged hiking trails, have been repaired and are open for business.

Lake Guntersville State Park is known across the South for its beautiful view of the lake itself. One of the more spectacular panoramas is from outside the lodge atop Taylor Mountain. You can take in even more impressive sights on the park's 36 miles of trail. One standout: Meredith Trail, which takes you to Town Creek, a lake tributary.

In addition to the lakeside views, the park is advertised as a "total recreation resort," and it lives up to that moniker. It has a hotel and chalets for those who don't like roughing it, as well as a restaurant and plenty to do. Within the park's boundaries there is an 18-hole championship golf course and a fishing center along Town Creek, which rents canoes and flat-bottomed boats. The park also offers beach swimming and, of course, those hiking trails.

One of the park's most popular events is Eagle Awareness Month. Every weekend in January, the park hosts conservation education programs and guided field trips to view bald eagles.

The park boasts 321 campsites. Seven modern bathhouses provide hot showers, and you will find coin-operated laundries in loops C and G.

:: Ratings

BEAUTY: ★ ★ ★ ★
PRIVACY: ★ ★ ★
SPACIOUSNESS: ★ ★ ★
QUIET: ★ ★ ★ ★
SECURITY: ★ ★ ★ ★
CLEANLINESS: ★ ★ ★ ★

:: Key Information

ADDRESS: 24 State Campground Rd., Guntersville, AL 35976	**FACILITIES:** Flush toilets, hot showers, playground, lake swimming, beach, camp store
OPERATED BY: Alabama State Parks	**PARKING:** At each site
CONTACT: 256-571-5455; 800-760-4108; alapark.com/lakeguntersville	**FEE:** Improved with water and power, $22; primitive, $13; add $5 for additional tent
OPEN: Year-round	
SITES: 321	**ELEVATION:** 614'
SITE AMENITIES: Improved–picnic table, fire ring with grill, water, power; Primitive–picnic table, fire ring	**RESTRICTIONS:**
	■ **Pets:** On leash only
ASSIGNMENT: First-come, first-serve or by reservation	■ **Fires:** In fire ring only
	■ **Alcohol:** Permitted
REGISTRATION: Pay attendant at office or by reservation	■ **Vehicles:** 2/site
	■ **Other:** Quiet hours 10 p.m.–6 a.m.

Each site has full amenities, including a barbecue grill, picnic table, water, and electricity. The sites have either level dirt or grass areas for tents. Several sites provide nice lake views. The best sites for views of the lake are in loop D, sites 7, 8, and 18; loop E, sites 8–11 and 35; and loop G, sites 11–12. A number of full-service sites provide not only water and power but sewer hook-ups for RVs as well. Even though you can pitch a tent there, they are the least desirable sites. These sites include all of loop B and F, as well as sites 12, 15, 17, 19, 21, 23–37, 39, 41, and 43 in loop G and sites 1–6 in loop H.

The excellent camp store has everything that you might have forgotten to pack, and let me tell you—the friendly attendants love to talk about their park.

Quarters are a little tight, which makes camping during summer and Eagle Awareness Month a bit cramped. Yes, even at limited capacity, this place teems with campers.

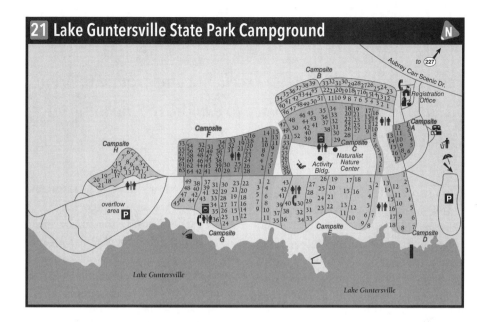

:: Getting There

From the intersection of US 431 and AL 227 in Guntersville, take AL 227 South 6 miles. Turn left onto Aubrey Carr Scenic Drive and travel 2.7 miles. Turn left onto State Campground Road. The country store where you register is 0.8 mile ahead on the left.

GPS COORDINATES   N34° 24.078'   W86° 12.229'

22

Mallard Creek Campground

"Very peaceful and quiet, an excellent campground to bring your family and a perfect place to explore the magnificent Wheeler National Wildlife Refuge"

This is one of my favorite Tennessee Valley Authority (TVA) campgrounds in Alabama. Sitting on a small finger of land jutting out into beautiful Wheeler Lake, Mallard Creek Campground offers peace and quiet. It's family-friendly and a perfect place to set up camp and explore the magnificent Wheeler National Wildlife Refuge.

Established in 1938, the refuge encompasses more than 35,000 acres of bottomland hardwoods, wetlands, and pine uplands that provide habitat for thousands of wintering waterfowl and migrating birds. The refuge hosts Alabama's largest duck population, plus 115 species of fish, 74 species of reptiles, 47 species of mammals, 285 species of songbirds, and 10 species of wildlife on the federal endangered or threatened lists. As the U.S. Fish and Wildlife Service puts it, Wheeler NWR provides a much-needed oasis for wildlife and migratory birds in what is ranked as one of the top 10 fastest-growing cities in the nation, Decatur. Mallard Creek Campground is only

:: Ratings

BEAUTY: ★ ★ ★ ★
PRIVACY: ★ ★ ★ ★
SPACIOUSNESS: ★ ★ ★ ★ ★
QUIET: ★ ★ ★ ★
SECURITY: ★ ★ ★ ★ ★
CLEANLINESS: ★ ★ ★ ★

a short 20-minute drive from the refuge's Givens Interpretative Center. Located off AL 67 east of Decatur, this 10,000-square-foot facility teaches about the area's amazing variety of wildlife. Visitors learn about animal habitats not only through displays but also first-hand in the center's Wildlife Observation Building.

This large, glass-enclosed room has bleachers and spotting scopes for viewing waterfowl and wading birds in an adjacent pond. The best time to view waterfowl is November–February. A backyard wildlife habitat behind the building has a waterfall and attracts many species of songbirds, butterflies, and hummingbirds. And a short 0.5-mile nature path, the Atkeson Cypress Trail, passes through a cypress swamp.

Admission to the visitor center is free. It's open March–September, Tuesday–Saturday, 9 a.m.–4 p.m.; and October–February, daily, 9 a.m.–5 p.m. For more information, contact the center at 256-350-6639.

Mallard Creek Campground has a single loop with 56 sites. You will find that all have plenty of elbowroom, so you are guaranteed privacy. The only exception might be sites 21 and 23–26, which are on a small road extending north from the main loop. One of the pleasures of Mallard Creek is that it is an exceptionally quiet campground.

Each site has gravel tent pads, power, water, a lantern post, a picnic table, and a

:: Key Information

ADDRESS: County Road 442, Decatur, AL 35603

OPERATED BY: Tennessee Valley Authority

CONTACT: 256-386-2560; tinyurl.com/tvacamp

OPEN: Mid-March–mid-November

SITES: 56

SITE AMENITIES: Improved–grass pad, picnic table, fire ring with grill, lantern post, water, power; Primitive–grass pad, picnic table, fire ring

ASSIGNMENT: First-come, first-serve

REGISTRATION: At camp manager's office

FACILITIES: Flush toilets, hot showers, playground, boat ramp, beach, fishing

PARKING: At each site

FEE: Improved with water and power, $22; primitive, $17

ELEVATION: 625'

RESTRICTIONS:

■ **Pets:** On leash

■ **Fires:** In fire ring or grill only; use deadfall or locally purchased wood

■ **Alcohol:** Prohibited

■ **Vehicles:** 2/site

■ **Other:** Quiet hours 10 p.m.–6 a.m.; 10 people/site; emergency contact TVA police 800-839-0003

fire ring with grill. And plenty of sites are along the waterfront. Most of the outer loop sites sit on the water. Sites 12, 16, and odd number sites 3–19 are on Mallard Creek, a lake tributary; sites 41, 43, and even number sites 28–50 are on Wheeler Lake itself. Hardwoods and pines offer decent shade during the hot summer months.

The bathhouse is next to the campground's main entrance, just past the gate. It's a heated, clean, medium-size facility with two hot showers, and it's handicap-accessible.

Register at the camp manager's office, just a few yards away from the entrance gate, which is locked after-hours. If you need to leave the campground when the gate is locked, contact the camp manager.

Like many other state and federal agencies that maintain and operate campgrounds and recreation areas, the TVA is concerned about the introduction of pests that can infest and kill trees. While we all agree it wouldn't be a campout without a roaring fire, bringing in your own outside firewood is the biggest cause of this problem. When camping, use only deadfall that you find around your campsite, or purchase wood locally.

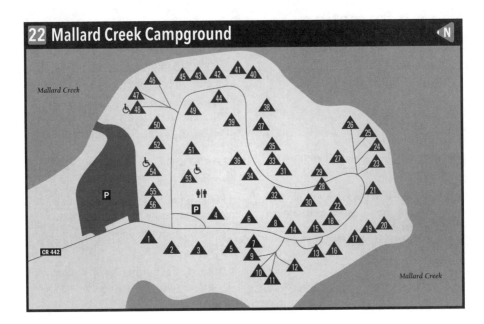

:: Getting There

From the intersection of County Road 67 and US 72/AL 20 West in Decatur, take US 72/AL 20 West 8.3 miles. Turn right onto Mallard Creek Road/CR 400. Travel 4 miles and turn right onto CR 442. Travel 0.2 mile. The camp host is on the left, and the campground entrance is to the right.

GPS COORDINATES　N34° 42.016'　W87° 09.519'

23

McFarland Park

"A perfect place to pitch camp and explore Southern living at its finest"

Located in the extreme northwest corner of the state, Florence is a beautiful, bustling burg, but not too big. On the banks of the Tennessee River, McFarland Park is a perfect location to pitch your tent and explore a city that is described as being "Southern living at its best." From beautiful high bluffs overlooking the majestic river to historic homes and outstanding outdoor activities, Florence and neighboring Muscle Shoals have something for everyone.

This part of the Tennessee River includes the Florence Fishing Trail, which consists of Pickwick, Wheeler, and Wilson Lakes. Trophy largemouth and smallmouth bass, crappie, and catfish are caught here along the grassy backwaters, shallows, and feeder streams either by boat or bank fishing.

Whether or not you have a boat, it's fascinating to watch the river traffic. And if you do have a boat, McFarland Park has an impressive 110-slip marina. It also features a floating two-story restaurant and bar, though the restaurant is open seasonally, so call ahead to check.

:: Ratings

BEAUTY: ★★★★
PRIVACY: ★★
SPACIOUSNESS: ★★
QUIET: ★★★
SECURITY: ★★★★
CLEANLINESS: ★★★★

If you're into festivals, there are two that you won't want to miss. The W. C. Handy Music Festival, held the last weekend of July, honors the man known as Alabama's Father of the Blues. The weekend features dozens of street parties, outdoor concerts, great food, and much more. It draws more than 150,000 people each year.

The other is the annual Frontier Days celebration. It's held the first full weekend of June and celebrates the region's heritage with period costumes, artisan demonstrations, food, and music. The event takes place at historic Pope's Tavern. Now a museum, the tavern was once a stagecoach stop and inn for passengers heading from Nashville to New Orleans in the 1800s. It's one of the city's oldest buildings.

And if you enjoy leisurely walks, be sure to take in one of the many walking tours of the city to soak up a little bit of the history and that Southern hospitality.

Across the river, you'll find the city of Muscle Shoals, where you can pay a visit to the Fame Recording Studio, the studio credited with starting the Southern rock sound, and Jack-o-Lantern Farm, a year-round farmers' market that offers hydroponically grown and naturally certified fruits and vegetables. The market is open Thursdays and Saturdays.

McFarland Park Campground offers 50 improved tent-camping sites and 6 primitive sites. The primitive sites dot the edge of

:: Key Information

ADDRESS: 200 James Spain Dr., Florence, AL 35630

OPERATED BY: City of Florence

CONTACT: 256-740-8817; tinyurl.com/mcfarlandcampground

OPEN: Year-round

SITES: 60 improved, 6 primitive

SITE AMENITIES: Improved–grass pad, picnic table, grill, water, power; Primitive–grass pad, picnic table, stone fire ring

ASSIGNMENT: First-come, first-serve or by reservation

REGISTRATION: At campground office or host site or by reservation

FACILITIES: Flush toilets, hot showers, laundry, playgrounds, fishing pier, driving range, soccer field, baseball field

PARKING: At each site

FEE: Improved, $14; primitive, $10; reservations require first night payment plus $3 reservation fee

ELEVATION: 447'

RESTRICTIONS:

■ **Pets:** On leash only; may require proof of vaccination; 2/site

■ **Fires:** In grill only; use only charcoal

■ **Alcohol:** Prohibited

■ **Vehicles:** 2/site

■ **Other:** Quiet hours 11 p.m.–6 a.m.; campground office open Monday–Saturday, 8 a.m.–9 p.m., and Sunday, noon–8 p.m.; 3-night minimum stay for Memorial Day, July 4, and Labor Day weekends; bike riding or skateboarding around bathhouse prohibited; clotheslines prohibited

the river and campground and include picnic tables and fire rings with level, grass tent pads. Improved sites include water, power, lantern post, and grills. The sites are very close together, leaving a lot to be desired for privacy and peace and quiet. Because the sites can accommodate either tents or RVs, each has its own large, paved parking strip. To pitch a tent use the narrow strip of grass next to the parking area.

The park and campground have many amenities. For the golfers there is a driving range; for the more team-sport oriented, there are soccer and baseball fields; and there's a lighted jogging trail that provides great views of the busy river and surrounding bluffs.

The campground has a single bathhouse with one hot shower. The bathhouse is medium-sized, very clean, and handicap-accessible. A coin-operated laundry occupies the rear of the bathhouse.

The campground is about 0.75 mile from the park entrance. The gate is locked at night, and Florence police patrol the park. The campground office, next to the entrance gate, is open April–September, 8 a.m.–5 p.m., and October–March, 1–5 p.m. If the office is closed when you arrive, see the camp host, whose RV is next to the office, to register.

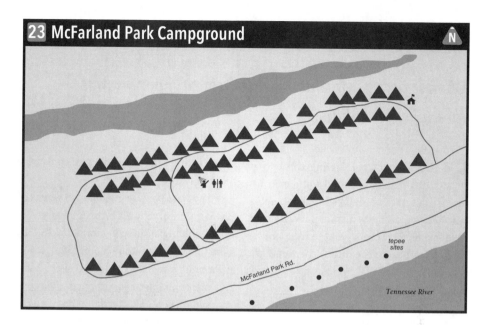

23 McFarland Park Campground

:: Getting There

From the intersection of Lee Highway/AL 13 and US 72 West/South Court Street in Florence, take US 72 West 0.5 mile and take the AL 20 exit. Travel 0.2 mile and merge left onto Coffee Road. Travel 0.2 mile and turn left onto McFarland Park Road. The campground entrance is 1.1 miles ahead.

GPS COORDINATES   N34° 46.895'   W87° 41.200'

24

Monte Sano State Park

"Change gears from suburbia to beautiful panoramas, waterfalls, and bluffs."

So there you are, driving through a suburban neighborhood with charming 1950s-era houses and oak-lined streets, and then you come to a state park. As you drive inside, the scenery suddenly changes from suburbia to beautiful panoramas, waterfalls, and bluffs. Welcome to Monte Sano State Park.

Monte Sano is on the east side of Huntsville, one of the fastest-growing cities in the state, in an area known as the Highland Rim. Thousands of years ago a vast ancient ocean covered this region. Over the millenniums the ocean began to recede and the land began to rise. Shell banks and coral reefs that once lined the ocean floor dried out, eventually forming the limestone bedrock that created this mountain.

Before its incarnation as a state park, Monte Sano was believed to have healing powers (Monte Sano is Spanish for "mountain of health"). In the early 1800s a hotel and sanitarium was built on top of the 1,600-foot peak and soon became a refuge for thousands of yellow fever victims who flocked to the mountain for the cool, crisp mountain air.

The state park opened in 1938 when the Civilian Conservation Corps (CCC) went to work, building an amazing infrastructure by hand that included stone cabins, a lodge, and an amphitheater. The CCC also constructed a network of hiking trails and picnic areas.

Since then, Monte Sano has been a favorite place for residents of north Alabama to take their children to hike the trails, teach them about nature, or hit the playground. Adults love to jog the trails or simply sit on a bluff and take in the wonderful views of deep hollows surrounded by rolling mountains. While spring–fall are the most popular seasons to visit, you will still find a good population of visitors and campers here in the winter as well.

If you plan on visiting, be sure to take in one of the many hiking and biking trails. The surrounding limestone bluffs make the treks both challenging and beautiful. Two of the best are the Stone Cuts Trail, a 3.5-mile out-and-back that takes you along towering limestone outcrops and through a narrow cave, and the MacKaye Hollow Trail that leads to the bottom of the hollow with amazing views, spring wildflowers, and a tumbling waterfall. And for mountain bikers, the Mountain Mist Trail is one of the finest you'll find in the area.

An added bonus is a trip to the Von Braun Observatory. The facility was built in

:: Ratings

BEAUTY: ★ ★ ★ ★
PRIVACY: ★ ★ ★
SPACIOUSNESS: ★ ★ ★
QUIET: ★ ★ ★ ★
SECURITY: ★ ★ ★ ★
CLEANLINESS: ★ ★ ★ ★

:: Key Information

ADDRESS: 5105 Nolen Ave., Huntsville, AL 35801

OPERATED BY: Alabama State Parks

CONTACT: 256-534-6589; alapark.com/montesano

OPEN: Year-round

SITES: 89 improved, 20 primitive

SITE AMENITIES: Improved–picnic table, fire ring with grill, water, power; Primitive–picnic table, fire ring, grill

ASSIGNMENT: First-come, first-serve or by reservation

REGISTRATION: Pay attendant at camp store or by reservation

FACILITIES: Flush toilets, hot showers, playground, camp store

PARKING: At each site

FEE: Improved with water, power, and sewer (for 4 people), $22 (Friday–Saturday, $25); improved with water and power (for 4 people), $19 (Friday–Saturday, $22); primitive (for 4 people), $13; add $2 for each additional person; add $5 for additional tent

ELEVATION: 437'

RESTRICTIONS:

■ **Pets:** On leash only

■ **Fires:** In fire ring or grill only

■ **Alcohol:** Prohibited

■ **Vehicles:** 2/site

■ **Other:** Quiet hours 10 p.m.–6 a.m.; 2 tents (8 people)/site

the late 1950s by Wernher Von Braun (this is the Rocket City, after all) and is used and maintained by the Von Braun Astronomical Society. Twice a month it opens the doors to the public for a planetarium show, sometimes a guest speaker such as a NASA astronaut, and then a walk outside to view the stars.

The campgrounds are some of the best around. Improved sites include a fire ring, a picnic table, water, and electricity. The tent pads are lined with fine gravel, or there is enough level, flat ground for pitching a tent. There is ample room for two cars in each site's paved driveway. Sites 3–11, 30, and 74–82 are reserved for RVs with full hook-ups.

The two bathhouses—one in the north loop, the other in the south loop—are spacious, clean, and heated, a welcome bonus for winter campers.

The 20 primitive sites are equally nice with level grassy tent pads, fire rings, and picnic tables. With plenty of room, you'll find peace and quiet.

Now it's no secret that I love to hike, and for me the best spots are in the primitive campground, sites 1–10. Just downhill from camp is the North Plateau Loop Trail, which leads directly to most all other trails in the park.

The well-stocked camp store at the entrance is where you will pay for your campsite. The campground is gated, providing adequate security. Campers get a code to exit the park after-hours.

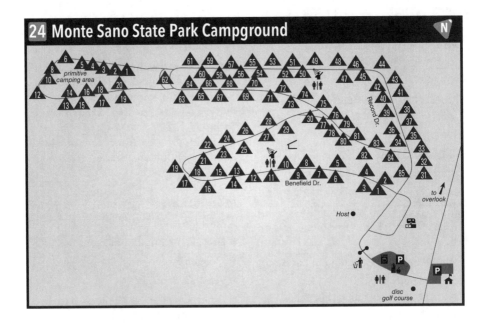

:: Getting There

From Huntsville take Governor's Drive SE/US 431 2.9 miles. Turn left onto Monte Sano Boulevard. Travel 2.4 miles and turn right onto Nolen Avenue SE. Travel 1.2 miles and make a sharp left onto Bankhead Parkway NE. Travel 0.2 mile and turn left. The entrance is on the right.

GPS COORDINATES N34° 44.630' W86° 30.719'

25

Noccalula Falls Campground

"Black Creek makes a spectacular 90-foot dive off a ledge atop Lookout Mountain into a natural gorge."

Several nice campgrounds in Alabama are operated by local municipalities, but one of my favorites is in Gadsden—the Noccalula Falls Campground.

The campground is actually a complex of three very popular entities—the campground, Noccalula Falls Miniature Golf Course, and Noccalula Falls Park. Each is operated and maintained by the city of Gadsden's Parks & Recreation department, and they are highly successful ventures.

The main draw is its namesake waterfalls. It is here that Black Creek makes a spectacular 90-foot dive off a ledge atop Lookout Mountain into a natural gorge.

The name comes from an old American Indian legend that dates to the time when the cascade was called Black Creek Falls. During that time, the daughter of a local Indian chief, Noccalula, was known throughout the region for her beauty and character. Many young braves wanted to marry her, but she was in love with a young man from her own tribe who lacked wealth. As is often the case in stories like this, her father had plans for her to marry a rich chief from a neighboring tribe.

Despite pleading with her father, the man she loved was driven out of the tribe and arrangements were made for her to wed the rich chief. On the day of the wedding, Noccalula dressed in her ceremonial attire and, overcome with grief, slipped away from the festivities and headed to the falls, the rushing water calling her. She made her way to the edge of the gorge and jumped. Distraught, her father changed the name of the waterfall to honor his daughter, and today a bronze statue of Noccalula stands at the edge of the chasm.

An interesting feature of the park is the Noccalula Falls Historic Hiking Trail. This difficult 1.4-mile loop leads down into the gorge. The first thing you will notice is the dramatic change in temperature. As you walk, the walls begin to tower above until you are face-to-face with the falls themselves. The trail leads directly behind the curtain of the waterfall.

Be very careful: The rocks are very slippery. Also stay away from the creek banks below the falls, where several visitors have drowned. Be sure to pick up a trail map and brochure at the entrance that indicate points of interest along the route.

Other park attractions include a pioneer village and railroad for the kids. Admission is $6 for adults, $4 for children ages 4–12, and free for children under age 4.

:: Ratings

BEAUTY: ★ ★ ★ ★
PRIVACY: ★ ★ ★ ★
SPACIOUSNESS: ★ ★ ★ ★
QUIET: ★ ★ ★ ★
SECURITY: ★ ★ ★ ★ ★
CLEANLINESS: ★ ★ ★ ★

:: Key Information

ADDRESS: 1600 Noccalula Rd., Gadsden, AL 35904

OPERATED BY: City of Gadsden

CONTACT: 256-543-7412; tinyurl.com/noccalula

OPEN: Year-round

SITES: 32

SITE AMENITIES: Grass pad, fire ring, some with grill, water, power

ASSIGNMENT: First-come, first-serve

REGISTRATION: At camp store

FACILITIES: Flush toilets, hot showers, laundry, pool, playground

PARKING: At each site

FEE: $16 (for 4 people); add $2 for each additional person

ELEVATION: 657'

RESTRICTIONS:

■ **Pets:** On leash only

■ **Fires:** In grill only

■ **Alcohol:** Prohibited

■ **Vehicles:** 1/site

■ **Other:** Quiet hours 10 p.m.–7 a.m.; 6 people/site

The miniature golf course is more than just your average putt-putt. Avid golfers will find this one a challenge. The course was laid out around natural geologic features with waterfalls and streams added to enhance the challenge. The course fee is $5 for adults and $4 for children age 12 and under.

The campground is exceptional to say the least. The first thing you'll notice when you spend a night here is the distant sound of the rushing water, which will lull you to sleep.

Unlike the park's 92 RV sites, which are a bit crowded, the tent-camping area provides ample space and plenty of shade from towering pines. Each site has water, power, and a fire ring. The tent pads are grass.

The bathhouse is just a short distance northeast of the tent sites. They are big, wide, and very clean. The facility is air-conditioned for those sticky summer days. It has four showers, one handicap-accessible. A coin-operated laundry, as well as an additional restroom, is available next to the park's office.

The park offers excellent security with a controlled entrance and exit gate, and the Gadsden police patrol the grounds.

The best times to pitch your tent at Noccalula are early spring and early fall, when the creek is at peak flow. If you center your trips on events, don't miss the annual Smoke on the Falls Barbecue Cook-off in mid-April or Christmas at the Falls from late November to December 23.

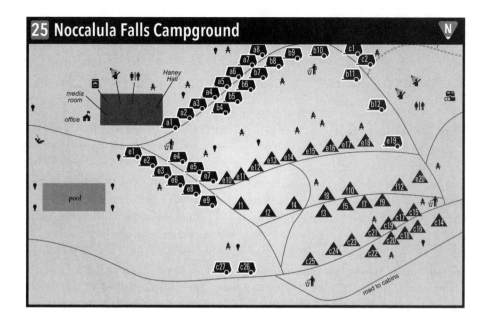

:: Getting There

From Gadsden take Broad Street 0.8 mile. Turn right onto North 12th Street. Travel 1.8 miles. The entrance will be on the left.

GPS COORDINATES   N34° 02.552'   W86° 01.319'

26

Rickwood Caverns State Park

"The perfect location to explore Alabama's underground world"

The old saying "beauty is only skin deep" does not apply to Alabama. Most state visitors see only Alabama's superficial beauty, what's on the surface—magnificent mountains, lakes, rivers, and streams. But another layer of natural beauty is beneath the surface, and Rickwood Caverns State Park is an ideal location to explore this underground realm, 175 feet underground to be precise.

Located midway between Huntsville and Birmingham in the town of Warrior, the park sits on an enormous limestone formation created some 250 million years ago. At that time a shallow ocean covered the region. Over the centuries, calcium from dying and decaying shell life was deposited on the ocean floor, eventually building into this massive crag.

The ocean receded over time, and as it did, water would percolate through the limestone, carving away at the rock and leaving thousands of caves behind. Alabama alone has more than 4,100 known caverns in this region. Even so, Rickwood stands out.

Although graffiti indicates that locals visited the cave as far back as the 1850s, it

:: Ratings

BEAUTY: ★ ★ ★ ★
PRIVACY: ★ ★ ★
SPACIOUSNESS: ★ ★ ★
QUIET: ★ ★ ★
SECURITY: ★ ★ ★
CLEANLINESS: ★ ★ ★

wasn't truly discovered until the 1950s, when a Boy Scout troop happened on it. The troop's leader, Eddie Rickles, began leading private cave tours until he sold the property in 1974, when it became a state park.

Taking one of the daily cave tours, you will immediately see why Rickwood is called the Miracle Mile. Turn after turn presents new and more breathtaking scenes. Passages are specially lighted to enhance the stalagmites and stalactites. Handrails provide balance as you meander through millions of years of geologic activity. But that activity is far from over. Walking the passages you will see water still dripping down the ancient columns, indicating that this is still a work in progress.

Along the route you will pass underground pools and might even see the rare blind cave fish. And don't forget to look at the ceiling as well. Evidence of the ancient ocean that once flowed can still be seen in the fossil remnants embedded above.

Keep in mind that you can only enter the cave with a guide. Tours are given weekends only March–Memorial Day and mid-August–October. Daily tours are given Memorial Day–mid-August. The cave is closed October–February.

Aside from the cave, visitors still find plenty to do here. You can take a dip in the park's Olympic-size swimming pool, which follows roughly the same schedule as the daily cave tours but stays open on weekends until Labor Day. You can also try your hand at mining for gems just like

:: Key Information

ADDRESS: 370 Rickwood Park Rd., Warrior, AL 35180

OPERATED BY: Alabama State Parks

CONTACT: 205-647-9692; alapark.com/rickwoodcaverns

OPEN: Year-round

SITES: 13 improved, 4 primitive

SITE AMENITIES: Improved sites–gravel pad, picnic table, fire ring with grate, water, power; Primitive–dirt/grass pad

ASSIGNMENT: First-come, first-serve

REGISTRATION: Pay at office

FACILITIES: Flush toilets, hot showers, pool, guided tours, snack bar

PARKING: At each site

FEE: Sunday-Thursday, $20.05 (for 4 people); Friday-Saturday, $23.05 (for 4 people); add $2 for each additional person; add $5 for additional tent (for children)

ELEVATION: 731'

RESTRICTIONS:

■ **Pets:** On leash only

■ **Fires:** In fire ring only; use only deadfall

■ **Alcohol:** Prohibited

■ **Vehicles:** 2/site

■ **Other:** Quiet hours 10 p.m.–6 a.m.; cave and pool open Memorial Day–mid-August, daily, and March–Memorial Day and mid-August–October, Saturday-Sunday, closed November–February

old-time prospectors at the Gemstone Mining Flume. Pick up a bag of mining dirt from the gift shop for $6. Or test your GPS skills by trying to locate one of the many geocaching spots (see the gift shop for details and policies). And take a hike along the Fossil Mountain Trail, a 1.2-mile loop passing through limestone boulders embedded with fossils. The park also has a small snack bar if you start craving something other than camp fare.

You will find camping at Rickwood Caverns State Park cozy. The improved campsites, 1–13, are rather close together, leaving a bit to be desired when it comes to privacy. There is also little shade along these sites. Each improved site has a compact crushed gravel pad, electricity, water, a picnic table, and a fire ring.

The four primitive campsites, on the other hand, are exceptional, spread far apart under a thick hardwood canopy that provides ample shade. The only drawback is that you are situated just downhill from Rickwood Caverns Road, and you will hear some car traffic from time to time, but since it is a lightly traveled road, the noise is not too disturbing.

While it's old, the bathhouse is nevertheless very clean and spacious. Each men's and women's side has two hot showers and is handicap-accessible. The bathhouses are unheated, but that's not a huge concern since most folks will visit the park during the spring and summer.

The main gate is locked at sunset. You will be provided with a number to call in case of emergencies after-hours.

26 Rickwood Caverns State Park

:: Getting There

From Birmingham take I-65 North 23.8 miles to Exit 284/US 31/AL 160 East/Hayden Corner. Turn left onto AL 160 West and travel 0.2 mile. Turn right onto Skyline Drive. Travel 2.5 miles and turn right onto Rickwood Caverns Road. Travel 1.9 miles to the park gate.

GPS COORDINATES   N33° 52.593'   W86° 51.887'

27

Slick Rock Campground

"The big draw to Slick Rock Campground is the fishing."

In northwest Alabama's Franklin County, visitors find four Tennessee Valley Authority (TVA) reservoirs, collectively known as Bear Creek Lakes. The four—Little Bear, Bear Creek (also called Big Bear), Upper Bear, and Cedar Creek—have a total of 8,280 surface acres of water providing remarkable and plentiful recreational activities.

The reservoirs were formed by flood-control dams built by the TVA in the late 1960s. They have served their purpose well but have the added attraction of offering many recreational opportunities, including fishing, boating, canoeing and kayaking, hiking, and camping.

Not long after the reservoirs were constructed, the Bear Creek Development Authority was formed to manage and maintain campgrounds and recreational areas around the lakes. Today the authority manages five campgrounds on 15,000 acres with 160 campsites.

Slick Rock Campground sits along the banks of Cedar Creek Reservoir, the largest of the four lakes with 4,200 surface acres of water. Now you would think that the reservoir is named for cedar trees. Well, not quite.

:: Ratings

BEAUTY: ★ ★ ★ ★
PRIVACY: ★ ★ ★ ★
SPACIOUSNESS: ★ ★ ★ ★
QUIET: ★ ★ ★ ★
SECURITY: ★ ★ ★ ★
CLEANLINESS: ★ ★ ★ ★

Early Europeans traveling and settling in the area mistook the region's many eastern juniper trees as cedars, and there you go.

An interesting side note about Cedar Creek is that at one time the area had an abundance of iron ore. Many years before the creek was dammed, it was the center of some very profitable mining operations. In fact, Cedar Creek Furnace led the state in iron manufacturing. The output was used for munitions during the Mexican and Civil Wars.

But the big draw for visitors now is the fishing. Anglers regularly haul in 5-, even 8-pound largemouth and spotted bass. The lake also has plentiful crappie, catfish, and threadfin shad. As always, an Alabama freshwater-fishing license is required.

The campground is only a short 10-mile drive from the town of Russellville, making this an excellent base for taking in the town's many activities and events; one of the biggest events is the Watermelon Festival. Held annually in the middle of August, the festival offers good old-fashioned family fun with an arts and crafts fair, scenic bike ride, 5K run, golf and tennis tournament, beauty pageant, antique car show, and, of course, plenty of watermelons.

After a day of eating watermelon and spending a hot summer afternoon at the festival, head back to camp for a welcome swim in the lake. The water is cool and the beach inviting. The beach is located between sites 20 and 21.

The campground sits on a thumb of land protruding from the lake's south bank.

:: Key Information

ADDRESS: Slick Rock Rd., Russellville, AL 35653

OPERATED BY: Bear Creek Development Authority

CONTACT: 877-367-2232; bearcreeklakes.com

OPEN: March–October

SITES: 53

SITE AMENITIES: Gravel pad, picnic table, grill, lantern post, water, power

ASSIGNMENT: First-come, first-serve

REGISTRATION: At camp store

FACILITIES: Flush toilets, hot showers, playground, boat ramp, lake swimming, beach, fishing pier, camp store

PARKING: At each site

FEE: $15

ELEVATION: 607'

RESTRICTIONS:

■ **Pets:** On leash only; not allowed in beach areas

■ **Fires:** In grill only

■ **Alcohol:** Prohibited

■ **Vehicles:** 2/site

■ **Other:** Quiet hours 11 p.m.–6 a.m.; 1 tent (8 people)/site; lanterns must be hung on provided posts

Eleven courtesy docks are found scattered around the perimeter of the peninsula.

In all, you'll find 53 sites in two loops at Slick Rock. The first loop includes sites 1–28 and loop two includes 29–53. Two sites, 27 and 28, are handicap-accessible. Each site has a gravel pad, water, power, a picnic table, a grill, and good shade provided by towering pines. There is ample spacing between each site, which guarantees plenty of privacy, plus the grounds themselves are very quiet. Of course since the campground is on a lake, the best sites are on the water. Sites 8, 9, 11, 13, 15–21, 40–42, and 45 are lakefront property.

Both campground loops have nice bathhouses that, although small, are big enough for the number of campers. The facilities are very clean with one hot shower. There is a playground and a camp store, where you will register and can pick up basic necessities.

The gate is locked at 10:30 p.m. Campers needing to leave or return after-hours should contact the on-duty ranger. The number will be provided upon registering.

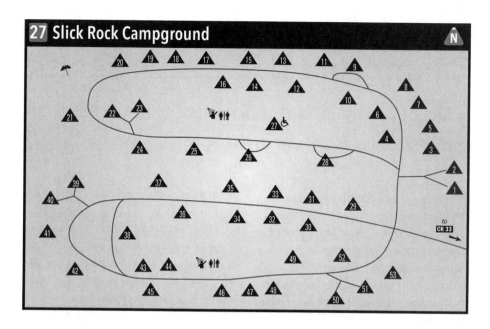

:: Getting There

From the intersection of East Lawrence Street and AL 24 West in Russellville, take AL 24 West 6.2 miles. Turn right onto AL 187 South. In 300 feet turn right onto County Road 524 and in another 300 feet turn left onto CR 49. Travel 2.7 miles and turn left onto CR 33. Travel 1.1 miles and turn right onto Slick Rock Campground Road. The camp store is on the right in 0.5 mile.

GPS COORDINATES N34° 30.663' W87° 54.588'

28

Wilson Dam–Lower Rockpile Campground

"A rustic campground with water access, premier bird-watching, and a great hiking trail"

On the banks of Pickwick Reservoir, just below the base of the Tennessee Valley Authority's Wilson Dam, you'll find a rustic little camping spot. The Wilson Dam–Lower Rockpile Campground, a self-service primitive facility, has only 23 sites, but what makes it special is the water access, premium bird-watching opportunities, and a great little hiking path, the Rockpile Trail.

The Rockpile Trail is a 6-mile, out-and-back National Recreational Trail. The well-maintained path follows the tall bluffs along the Tennessee River and is marked with white blazes. The hike is considered moderately strenuous because of the hills.

The trail offers some nice views of the city of Florence and a remarkable variety of birds. Along the route you're apt to see pelicans, Baltimore orioles (not the baseball team), great crested flycatchers, blue herons, ospreys, any number of other waterfowl and gulls, and on and on and on. For a complete list, visit the North Alabama

Birding Trail website: **northalabamabirding trail.com**.

You'll find some pretty impressive landscapes along the route as well, such as several small caves and a cascading waterfall near the base of Wilson Dam. And you'll have a chance to experience plenty of history along the route too, as it passes the old foundations of the Wilson Steam Plant that was once the largest such facility in the world; a beautiful stone Civilian Conservation Corps picnic pavilion overlooking the river; and two Civil War earthworks built by General John Bell Hood and his troops.

The 50-mile-long Pickwick Reservoir stretches from the Pickwick Landing Dam in Tennessee to Wilson Dam in Florence, with a total surface area of more than 47,000 acres. Fishing is excellent, with the main catches being largemouth and smallmouth bass. There is a 14-inch minimum size restriction on your catch. The fishing is so good here that several line records (the size of the fishing line used to make the catch) were set here. Visitors find a fishing pier and boat ramp at the western end of the campground.

But the Wilson Dam–Lower Rockpile Campground is a rustic, primitive campground with not much in the way of amenities, so be sure to bring what you need for your stay. The sites line up from east to west, and all but sites 4, 6, 8, 9, 11–14 are along the

:: Ratings

BEAUTY: ★ ★ ★
PRIVACY: ★ ★ ★
SPACIOUSNESS: ★ ★ ★ ★
QUIET: ★ ★ ★ ★
SECURITY: ★ ★ ★
CLEANLINESS: ★ ★

:: Key Information

ADDRESS: Reservation Rd., Muscle Shoals, AL 35633

OPERATED BY: Tennessee Valley Authority

CONTACT: 800-882-5263; tinyurl.com/tvacamp

OPEN: Year-round

SITES: 23

SITE AMENITIES: Picnic table, stone fire ring, grill, trash cans

ASSIGNMENT: First-come, first-serve

REGISTRATION: At self-pay kiosk (cash only)

FACILITIES: Flush toilets, hot showers, boat ramp, fishing pier

PARKING: At each site

FEE: $17

ELEVATION: 398'

RESTRICTIONS:

■ **Pets:** On leash only

■ **Fires:** In grills or fire ring only; use only deadfall or locally purchased wood

■ **Alcohol:** Prohibited

■ **Vehicles:** 2/site

■ **Other:** Quiet hours 10 p.m.–6 a.m.; 4 people/site

banks of the reservoir. If you like bank fishing, you'll love these. The best with water views are sites 15–23. The others have a narrow treeline partially blocking the water. All the sites are very level with the exception of site 10, which has a bit of a slope to it.

Site amenities include a gravel or dirt tent pad, picnic table, stone fire ring, and trash can. You'll find the bathhouse between sites 9 and 11. It's rather old and tends to be dirty, but it has hot showers and, compared to the state's other primitive sites, is really pretty nice.

Wilson Dam–Lower Rockpile Campground is a self-service campsite, which means that you pay as you enter. As you drive down to the reservoir, you will pass sites 19–23 to the left (north) as well as a large parking area for boaters, the fishing

pier, and the boat ramp. Soon you will come to a pipe fence. The pay station is on the right side of the fence. Simply complete the information on the outside of the provided envelopes, put your cash inside, and then drop it into the kiosk, making sure to keep the registration tag for your car to prove that you paid. The TVA asks that you pay on a daily basis instead of for multiple days at a time because it cannot provide refunds if you leave early.

The campground does not have a locked gate but is patrolled regularly by TVA guards.

As you enter the campground make sure to note the FALLING ROCKS warning sign at the entrance gate. The tall bluff along the road could drop some rocks, so don't linger by the cliff and keep your head up.

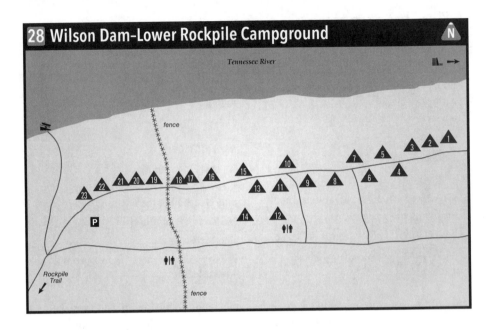

:: Getting There

From the intersection of US 72 and AL 133/South Cox Creek Road in Florence, take AL 133 South 2.6 miles. After crossing Wilson Dam, continue 0.5 mile and turn right (look for the Wilson Dam–Lower Rockpile sign). In about 0.5 mile the road bends to the right and leads to the campground entrance.

GPS COORDINATES N34° 47.522' W87° 38.121'

River Region

29

Blue Springs State Park

"Well worth spending a night or two to enjoy the peace and serenity and a gorgeous blue spring"

At only 103 acres, Blue Springs State Park is one of Alabama's smallest state parks, but it's well worth the time to visit and spend a night or two and enjoy the peaceful and serene campground and a gorgeous blue spring.

Located in the small town of Clio in Barbour County, Blue Springs State Park offers peace and quiet and the opportunity to do something you can't do in most states—take a dip in a natural spring. Nature pumps up to 3,600 gallons of crystal-clear water per minute into the pond and maintains a constant temperature of 68°F. Beneath the deep-blue waters is a sandy bottom, and as you gaze into it you'll see some pretty good-size fish swimming about.

The property was originally owned by J. D. McLaughlin. In 1963 the state purchased the land and immediately began work on developing it into a park. The pond was divided into two sections with the creation of a 2-foot-wide cement wall around the perimeter. This was then bisected with a cement bridge. The bridge has an archway that allows the water to flow from one side to the other and then flow out into the Choctawhatchee River, which also flows through the park. Stairs lead down into the pond, so you can actually swim in it, a blessing on one of the hot, humid summer days of the South. Remember, there is no lifeguard on duty and swimming is at your own risk.

The Choctawhatchee River flows through the park and has its headwaters nearby. This narrow stream eventually widens and deepens as it winds more than 140 miles into Florida and eventually the Gulf of Mexico. The river is considered one of Alabama's 10 natural wonders. A walk along the banks just below the spring's spillway passes under tall oaks draped in Spanish moss.

The park also has a large fishing pond, which is closed on Monday (except on holidays) and Tuesday. The lake is abuzz in late May each year as it hosts a Youth Fishing Rodeo. The water is fully stocked for young anglers trying to win prizes, and park admission is waived. Contact the park for dates and times. Remember that an Alabama freshwater-fishing license is required.

If you enjoy attending festivals, then check out the annual Brundidge Peanut Butter Festival, held annually the last weekend of October. In the 1930s the town had a thriving peanut butter industry. Today that heritage is celebrated with this festival featuring arts and crafts and peanuts of all types—boiled, roasted, parched—you name it, they'll have it. Contact the city at 334-735-3125 for information.

:: Ratings

BEAUTY: ★ ★ ★ ★ ★
PRIVACY: ★ ★ ★
SPACIOUSNESS: ★ ★ ★
QUIET: ★ ★ ★ ★
SECURITY: ★ ★ ★ ★
CLEANLINESS: ★ ★ ★ ★

:: Key Information

ADDRESS: 2595 AL 10, Clio, AL 36017

OPERATED BY: Alabama State Parks

CONTACT: 334-397-4875;
alapark.com/bluesprings

OPEN: Year-round

SITES: 50

SITE AMENITIES: Improved—gravel pad, picnic table, fire ring with grate, water, power; Primitive—grass pad, picnic table, fire ring

ASSIGNMENT: First-come, first-serve

REGISTRATION: At office at the park's entrance

FACILITIES: Flush toilets, hot showers, playground, natural spring, fishing

PARKING: At each site

FEE: Improved (for 4 people/Sunday–Thursday), $19.76; improved (for 4 people/Friday–Saturday), $22.88; primitive, $13.52; add $2 for each additional person; add $5 for additional tent (for children)

ELEVATION: 353'

RESTRICTIONS:

■ **Pets:** On leash only

■ **Fires:** In fire ring only; use only deadfall

■ **Alcohol:** Prohibited

■ **Vehicles:** 1/site

■ **Other:** Quiet hours 10 p.m.–6 a.m.; 1 tent (8 people)/site, extra tent for children allowed

Blue Springs State Park has two playgrounds, along with a ball field and a volleyball court. You'll find 50 improved campsites and an open area for primitive camping at the park. Each improved site has compact crushed gravel pads, water, electricity, a fire ring with a grate for cooking, and a picnic table. The primitive spots have fire rings and picnic tables. There are no assigned sites in the primitive area. To access it, look for the dirt road off the main campground road to your right between improved sites 8 and 9. This road leads you to the primitive camp area and also loops around to the bathhouse.

The improved campsites are a bit close together, so you lose a little in privacy, but overall most sites are very nice and shady under the big hardwoods, most notably sites 18–35. Sites 22 and 23 are near the river.

The one heated bathhouse sits between the improved and primitive loops. It's very clean and handicap-accessible, and it has three hot showers.

The front gate is locked at 7 p.m. in the summer, at 6 p.m. in March, April, October, and November, and at 5 p.m. December–February. If you need assistance after-hours, the park manager's house is next to the entrance gate.

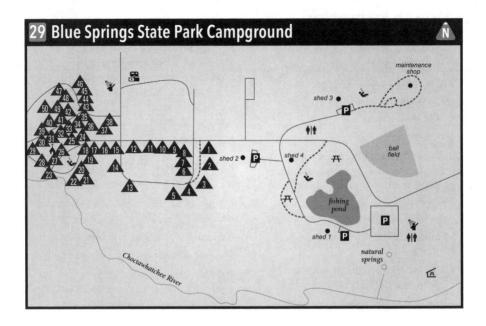

:: Getting There

From Troy take AL 10 East 29.7 miles. The entrance is on the left.

GPS COORDINATES   N31° 39.823'   W85° 30.458'

30

Bluff Creek Campground

"Bluff Creek Campground features waterfront sites plus fantastic views and cool lake breezes."

The best US Army Corps of Engineers property has to be Bluff Creek Campground, which features waterfront sites plus fantastic views and cool lake breezes. Located on the banks of Walter F. George Lake and two reservoir tributaries, Bluff Creek and Mill Creek, almost every site is right on the water.

The history of the Corps of Engineers can be traced to 1775, when the Continental Congress organized an army of engineers led by Colonel Richard Gridley. Eventually this new army played key roles in major Revolutionary War battles, including Bunker Hill and Yorktown. It wasn't until 1802 that the Corps of Engineers' mission was set in stone—to contribute to military construction and "works of a civil nature." In Alabama that mission is significant, considering the thousands of miles of rivers that course through the state. The Corps' projects provide hydroelectric power and flood control to the area, as well as recreational activities, such as this beautiful campground.

:: Ratings

> **BEAUTY:** ★ ★ ★ ★
> **PRIVACY:** ★ ★ ★
> **SPACIOUSNESS:** ★ ★ ★
> **QUIET:** ★ ★ ★ ★
> **SECURITY:** ★ ★ ★ ★ ★
> **CLEANLINESS:** ★ ★ ★ ★

As mentioned elsewhere, the Chattahoochee begins as a tumbling, turbulent spring-fed stream in north Georgia. Over the centuries the river has provided drinking water, irrigation for the region's fertile farmland, and more. In the past 20 years the river has been the center of what has become known as the Water War.

The river flows near the burgeoning city of Atlanta, supplying its residents with their water needs to the tune of 400 million gallons a day. The states of Alabama and Florida are concerned that the draining of the reservoir near Atlanta could significantly impact the health, well-being, and economy of towns and cities downstream and have filed several federal lawsuits to protect the river. The issue is still being fought in the courts today.

While the war wages on, people flock to the area for the bountiful recreational activities on this beautiful river. Amazing fishing is among the activities that you can enjoy here along the banks of the Chattahoochee and Bluff Creek. Cast your line for largemouth and white bass, crappie, channel catfish, and bream. For birders, Bluff Creek Campground offers the opportunity to spot bald eagles, waterfowl of all types (including wood ducks and Canada geese), red-tailed hawks, and an astonishing array of songbirds. And don't forget wildlife spotting. On any given day you can see white-tailed deer and bobcats.

:: Key Information

ADDRESS: 144 Bluff Creek Rd., Pittsview, AL 36871

OPERATED BY: US Army Corps of Engineers

CONTACT: 334-855-2746; reservations 877-444-6777; tinyurl.com/bluffcreek

OPEN: March–October

SITES: 88

SITE AMENITIES: Gravel pad, picnic table, fire ring, water, power; Mill Run also has lantern posts and a prep table; River Forest also has grills

ASSIGNMENT: First-come, first-serve or by reservation

REGISTRATION: At entry gate or by reservation

FACILITIES: Flush toilets, hot showers, laundry, playground, boat launch, lake swimming, fishing, fish-cleaning station

PARKING: At each site; additional parking inside Mill Run, River Forest, and Pine Bluff Loops across from campsites

FEE: $20

ELEVATION: 215'

RESTRICTIONS:

■ **Pets:** On leash only; not allowed in beach areas, playgrounds, or restrooms

■ **Fires:** In fire ring or grill only; use only deadfall

■ **Alcohol:** Prohibited

■ **Vehicles:** 3/site

■ **Other:** Quiet hours 10 p.m.–6 a.m.; 8 people/site; must obtain pass and display in windshield before entering; 2-night minimum stay on weekends; 3-night minimum stay on holidays

Once again the Corps of Engineers has outdone itself with this campground. The campground has five loops: the Uchee Trail Loop with sites 1–10, Mill Run with 11–19, River Forest with 20–51, Pine Bluff with 52–70, and Cherokee Loop with 71–88. Sites 1–26, 48–58, and 71–88 can be reserved, but the remainder are strictly first-come, first-serve.

While the number of waterfront spots makes this a very attractive and popular campground, the sites tend to be rather close together, so you lose a little peace, quiet, and privacy, but it's nothing unbearable.

Each loop offers different amenities. The sites are all improved with compact crushed gravel pads, water, electricity, a fire ring, and a picnic table. The Mill Run Loop also has lantern posts and a prep table. River Forest has the addition of grills. While all campsites have their own cement driveway for parking, additional parking is scattered around

the campground. These will be found across from sites 5–7, 15–17, 27–31, and 63.

The campground features three spacious bathhouses, each well maintained, very clean, and handicap-accessible. Each men's and women's side has two hot showers. A nice touch is that each one also has its own coin-operated laundry.

As mentioned earlier, Bluff Creek has excellent fishing, and the Corps of Engineers serves anglers with a nice cement boat launch and a fish-cleaning station, complete with running water, near the campground entrance. For the kids, a great little playground can be found in the Pine Bluff Loop.

Security is excellent here, as with all Corps of Engineers sites. The entrance at the park attendant's station has gates that are locked after-hours, and the camp hosts, all very friendly and informative, live near the entrance for your convenience and security.

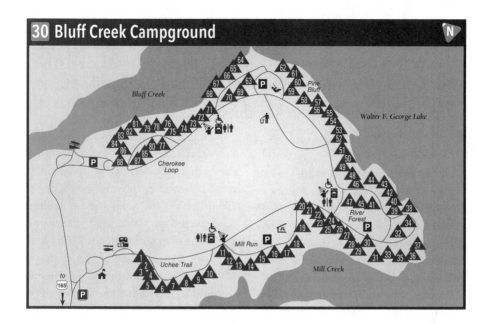

:: Getting There

From Pittsview travel east on Pecan Street 0.9 mile. Turn right onto County Road 4. Travel 6.4 miles. Turn left onto AL 165 North. Travel 4.1 miles. Turn right onto Bluff Creek Road. The entrance is 1 mile ahead on the right.

GPS COORDINATES   N32° 11.159'   W85° 00.830'

31

Chewacla State Park

"The 30-foot Chewacla Falls is an impressive cascade formed by the spillway of Chewacla Dam."

For many years I had heard about Chewacla State Park from hiking and outdoorsy friends but never had a chance to visit. I figured that it was just another small state park and couldn't be that special. I finally made the trip, and brother, was I wrong. Although relatively small at 695 acres, the park offers plenty of recreational opportunities and a great camping experience.

On the outskirts of the bustling college town of Auburn, Chewacla was built in the 1930s by the Civilian Conservation Corps (CCC). As is the case in many Alabama state parks, evidence of the young men's craftsmanship can be seen in the stone masonry of the hand-built structures that still stand today and are even now used as cabins for lodging. A stout old CCC bridge with beautiful locally mined hand-laid stones forms the structure's single archway.

On the recreational side, the standout attraction is the park's hiking trails. The eight trails total more than 7 miles and range in difficulty from easy to moderate. Along the web of trails you might see red foxes, white-tailed deer, and turkeys.

One of the most popular paths is the Mountain Laurel Trail. It takes visitors to the 30-foot Chewacla Falls, an impressive cascade formed by the spillway of Chewacla Dam. There is also a popular 2-mile single-track mountain biking trail that is rated beginning to intermediate in difficulty.

Speaking of biking, if you enjoy two-wheeled touring, be sure to visit Chewacla in mid-May for the Alabama Magnificent Bicycling Adventure. Pitch camp in the park for the week and enjoy a new bike ride along historic loops each day. Proceeds from the event help support AlaBike, a nonprofit organization dedicated to making the state a better, and safer, place to ride bikes.

Other park amenities include a swimming beach on the banks of the 26-acre Chewacla Lake. The lake is also great for canoeing and kayaking (canoes are available for rent, as are pedal boats) and has excellent fishing. An Alabama freshwater-fishing license is required.

The park affords excellent tent camping as well. The improved sites are divided into two loops. McVay Loop includes sites 1–16, while the Watts Loop includes 17–36. Between the two loops are 10 primitive campsites, all shaded under a canopy of pines and hardwoods. The improved sites have compact crushed gravel pads, power, water, a picnic table, and a fire ring with grate. Primitive sites have compact crushed gravel pads as well as fire rings. By the way, firewood is available for sale at the park entrance; otherwise use deadfall for your campfires. The

:: Ratings

BEAUTY: ★ ★ ★ ★
PRIVACY: ★ ★ ★ ★
SPACIOUSNESS: ★ ★ ★ ★
QUIET: ★ ★ ★
SECURITY: ★ ★ ★ ★
CLEANLINESS: ★ ★ ★ ★

:: Key Information

ADDRESS: 124 Shell Toomer Pkwy., Auburn, AL 36830

OPERATED BY: Alabama State Parks

CONTACT: 344-887-5621; reservations 800-272-7275; alapark.com/chewacla

OPEN: Year-round

SITES: 46

SITE AMENITIES: Improved—gravel pad, picnic table, fire ring with grate, water, power; Primitive—fire ring with grate

ASSIGNMENT: First-come, first-serve or by reservation (no reservations taken for primitive sites)

REGISTRATION: At camp store or by reservation

FACILITIES: Flush toilets, hot showers, laundry, lake swimming, beach, fishing

PARKING: At each site

FEE: Improved with water and power, August–November, Sunday–Thursday, $25 (Friday–Saturday, $28); improved with water and power, December–July, $19 (March–July, Friday–Saturday, $22); primitive, $13; add $6 for additional tent (for children)

ELEVATION: 510'

RESTRICTIONS:

■ **Pets:** On leash only; not allowed on beach or in park buildings

■ **Fires:** In fire ring only; use only deadfall or purchase wood at office

■ **Alcohol:** Prohibited

■ **Vehicles:** 2/site

■ **Other:** Quiet hours 10 p.m.–6 a.m.; 2-night minimum stay on weekends; 3-night minimum stay on holidays; 1 tent (4 people)/site

store also has a limited amount of supplies that you might have forgotten.

There are two bathhouses, one inside the McVay Loop and the other in the Watts Loop. Both are rather small but are very clean with hot showers. The heated facilities are also handicap-accessible. The Watts Loop facility has a coin-operated laundry.

The kids will enjoy the playground on the banks of Chewacla Lake, located north of the campgrounds across the camp road. The lake also provides fishing and swimming opportunities. When swimming, remember that no lifeguards are on duty, so use caution.

Now here's the bad news. Being so close to Auburn University means that your chances of getting a campsite during a football home-game weekend will be tough. Most campers make their reservations well in advance (probably as soon as the ink has dried on the Southeastern Conference football schedule), and the park does not take reservations for the primitive sites—those are strictly first-come, first-serve. You can reserve an improved site by calling the number in the sidebar above. Reservations require a two-night minimum stay, which must be paid in advance.

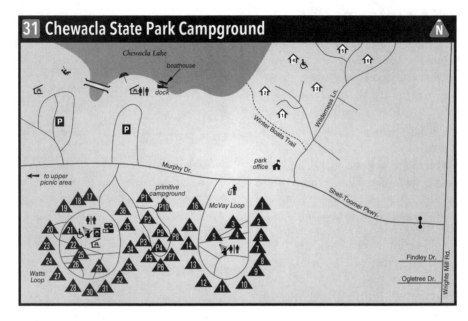

:: Getting There

From Auburn take AL 15 South/North College Street 4.3 miles. Turn left onto CR 674/Shell Toomer Parkway. Travel 1.5 miles to the park entrance.

GPS COORDINATES   N32° 33.240'   W85° 28.810'

32

Chilatchee Creek Campground

"Thick, flowing Spanish moss draped like curtains from towering oaks, a scene yanked right out of the pages of Gone with the Wind"

Thick, flowing Spanish moss draped like curtains from towering oaks greeted me like a scene yanked from the pages of *Gone with the Wind* as I drove into Chilatchee Creek Campground for my first visit.

Of all of the US Army Corps of Engineers campgrounds I have visited, this one was different. While all Corps campgrounds are relatively quiet, this one is exceptionally quiet! In fact, as you pull up to the gate, the camp host may proudly proclaim, "Hope you like it quiet. We've got a lot of that."

Chilatchee is one of the smaller Corps of Engineers properties. Combine that with its out-of-the-way location in Wilcox County, and you can see why this hushed oasis in southwest Alabama makes it one of the best getaway campouts you'll have.

The Chilatchee Creek Campground is located on its namesake creek that feeds the larger Dannelly Reservoir. The 27-square-mile reservoir is the product of the Millers Ferry Lock and Dam several miles

downriver. In all, Dannelly has more than 500 miles of shoreline.

The Alabama River is the backbone of the region, providing a route for commerce to the Gulf of Mexico and recreational opportunities for locals and visitors.

The waters also have made this region some of the most fertile farming land anywhere. The layers of dark, rich soil deposited over the centuries make this area of the Black Belt excellent for growing cotton, wheat, and, with proper irrigation, even rice.

The region, especially here in Wilcox County, has seen its share of hard times, but the small, close-knit communities have held together through the good and the bad. One of their biggest success stories, and one that has given them world acclaim, is the beautiful quilt tapestries that the residents create. The art has been passed down from generation to generation and began mostly out of necessity for cold winters, but of late has continued as an American art form. The Gee's Bend quilters meet to practice their art Monday–Thursday, 8:30 a.m.–1:30 p.m. (times may vary), at the nearby Boykin Nutrition Center. Visitors (and shoppers) are welcome.

Chilatchee is an American Indian word, believed to be Choctaw in origin, that means "fox river." Yes, there is a good chance that

:: Ratings

BEAUTY: ★ ★ ★ ★ ★
PRIVACY: ★ ★ ★
SPACIOUSNESS: ★ ★ ★ ★
QUIET: ★ ★ ★ ★
SECURITY: ★ ★ ★ ★ ★
CLEANLINESS: ★ ★ ★ ★

:: Key Information

ADDRESS: 2267 Chilatchee Creek Rd., Alberta, AL 36720

OPERATED BY: US Army Corps of Engineers

CONTACT: 334-573-2562; reservations 877-444-6777; tinyurl.com/chilatchee

OPEN: Improved, March–early September; Primitive, year-round

SITES: 53

SITE AMENITIES: Improved–gravel pads, picnic table, fire ring, grill, lantern post, water, power; Primitive–grass pads, fire ring, grill

ASSIGNMENT: First-come, first-serve or by reservation

REGISTRATION: At entry gate or by reservation

FACILITIES: Flush toilets, hot showers, laundry, fishing, playground, fish-cleaning station, courtesy docks

PARKING: At each site

FEE: Waterfront sites, $20; non-waterfront sites, $18; primitive, $14

ELEVATION: 97'

RESTRICTIONS:

■ **Pets:** On leash only; not allowed in restrooms or playgrounds

■ **Fires:** In fire ring or grill only; use only deadfall

■ **Alcohol:** Prohibited

■ **Vehicles:** 3/site

■ **Other:** Quiet hours 10 p.m.–6 a.m.; 8 people/site; must obtain pass and display in windshield before entering

you will catch a glimpse of a fox or two here, as well wild turkeys, bobcats, coyotes, and white-tailed deer. And alligators are in the area too, so keep your distance.

If you are a boater of any kind, whether you like to canoe or kayak with a paddle, drop in a trolling motor, or have a small runabout, you will appreciate the courtesy docks here. Six such docks are available between sites 9 and 10, 11 and 12, 15 and 16, 20 and 21, and 29 and 30. One additional dock is located on a spit of land extending north into the creek next to a picnic shelter. And the docks aren't just for boats. They are great places to sit and watch a sunrise or sunset. A cement boat launch is here as well.

If you want a view of the water (and who wouldn't?), sites 9–24 front the creek and provide breathtaking views.

All improved sites have compact crushed gravel pads, power, water, a picnic table, and a lantern post. Primitive sites have grass tent pads, a fire ring, a grill, and a picnic table. These sites, 48–53, are located just inside the gate behind the camp host. Best of all, every site has plenty of shade courtesy of those magnificent hardwoods.

The campground has a single bath-house, but it is more than adequate for the size of the park and the number of people who visit. The facility has a unique design. The northeast side has spacious men's and women's restrooms. The southwest side has three hot showers—a men's, women's, and handicapped. The showers are actually individual rooms. Once again, the facility is well maintained and clean.

As you arrive on Chilatchee Park Road, you will notice that the first mile is dirt and gravel before it becomes pavement again for the remaining drive to the entrance. Just after turning onto Chilatchee Creek Road,

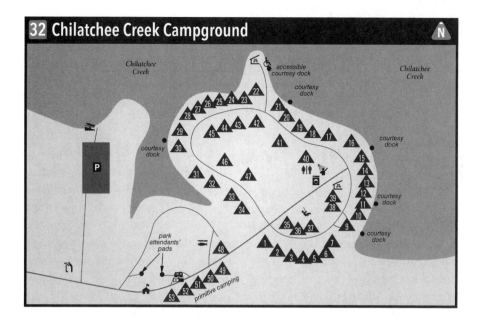

there is a scenic overview where you can stop and try to take a look at the creek from atop a bluff. When I visited, the brush had grown up, so I couldn't see the view. Perhaps in the fall when the leaves are gone, you can take in the vista.

:: Getting There

From Selma take AL 22 West 23.4 miles. Bear left onto AL 5 South/Jefferson Davis Highway. Travel 4.7 miles, and turn left onto CR 29. Travel 8.6 miles, and turn left onto Chilatchee Park Road. Travel 1.1 miles and turn left onto Chilatchee Creek Road. The park entrance is ahead in 0.5 mile.

GPS COORDINATES   N32° 08.460'   W87° 16.423'

33

Fort Toulouse–Fort Jackson National Historic Park

"More than 6,000 years of history await you."

More than 6,000 years of history await you at the Fort Toulouse–Fort Jackson National Historic Park. Located at the headwaters of the Alabama River, at the confluence of the Tallapoosa and Coosa Rivers, the area was first inhabited by nomadic hunters circa 5000 B.C., with the first true settlement established by the American Indians of the Mississippian period circa 1000 A.D. These settlers built ceremonial and residential mounds in this area.

In 1540 Hernando de Soto became the first European to explore the area. In the early 1700s, the region was split between France and Britain. The French feared a British takeover and built a fort here because they believed the site was the most valuable strategic position in the Southeast. They named it after the son of King Louis XIV, Count de Toulouse.

In 1740 the fort was in desperate need of repair, and the French invested a considerable amount of money to rebuild it just south of its original location.

Following their defeat in the French and Indian War of 1763, France turned control of

:: Ratings

BEAUTY: ★ ★ ★ ★
PRIVACY: ★ ★ ★
SPACIOUSNESS: ★ ★ ★
QUIET: ★ ★ ★ ★
SECURITY: ★ ★ ★ ★
CLEANLINESS: ★ ★ ★ ★

the fort over to the British, but the new caretakers never really manned or maintained it, and by 1776 it had once again fallen into disrepair and succumbed to Mother Nature.

Years later, General Andrew Jackson began rebuilding on the site of the original fort. In the summer of 1814 Jackson won a decisive battle against the Creek people at Horseshoe Bend, which effectively ended the Creek Indian War. The resulting treaty was signed here at what was then called Fort Jackson.

Shortly after the treaty signing, the fort became the first seat of Montgomery County. But once again, it began to decline, this time from the migration of residents to the state's new capital, Montgomery. By 1819 the town was left to be reclaimed by nature.

In 1971 the Alabama Historic Commission acquired the property, and archeological work began to uncover the history of Fort Toulouse–Fort Jackson. Now it's the site of an impressive archeological park.

The park hosts living history weekends throughout the year, depicting fort life from its earliest days to the last of the European influences. Be sure to visit the Grave's House Visitor Center and Museum. Not only do you pay your camping fees here but you can also take a look at an interesting collection of French Colonial, early American, and American Indian artifacts.

Hikers will find a short interpretive path, the William Bartram Arboretum

:: Key Information

ADDRESS: 2521 West Fort Toulouse Rd., Wetumpka, AL 36093

OPERATED BY: Alabama Historic Commission

CONTACT: 334-567-3002; forttoulouse.com

OPEN: Year-round; closed January 1, Thanksgiving, and December 25

SITES: 39

SITE AMENITIES: Dirt tent pad, picnic table, grill, water, power

ASSIGNMENT: First-come, first-serve

REGISTRATION: Pay attendant at office or by reservation

FACILITIES: Flush toilets, hot showers, playground, boat ramp, camp store, museum

PARKING: Limited to the number that fit on paved drive available at each campsite; additional parking at bathhouse

FEE: $12; add $8 for additional tent

ELEVATION: 178'

RESTRICTIONS:

■ **Pets:** On leash only

■ **Fires:** In fire ring or grill only; use only deadfall

■ **Alcohol:** Permitted

■ **Vehicles:** Limited to the number that fit on paved drive at campsite, at least 2

■ **Other:** Quiet hours 9 p.m.–7 a.m.; 3 tents (8 people)/site; gates locked at 9 p.m.

Trail, named after the 18th-century botanist who explored this area. The trail leads through beautiful hardwood forests over boardwalks and dirt paths. And be sure to take a look at the views of the river from the park's high bluffs.

The campground sites are wide and spacious. All 39 are improved with water, electricity, grills, and picnic tables. All but sites 4–6 are available for tent camping.

Fort Toulouse is one of the few sites that allows up to three tents on one site. The $12 fee is for one tent. You'll pay $8 extra for each additional tent. Parking is limited to the number of vehicles that can fit on the site's paved parking area. Additional parking is available at the bathhouse.

And speaking of which, the bathhouse is very nice: big and spacious, very clean, and heated for those cold winter months.

You can reserve a campsite in advance, but you are only assured of a spot, not a specific site. When you arrive you will pass the campground on your right and continue straight for about 0.1 mile to the visitor center, where you will pay for your site.

33 Fort Toulouse–Fort Jackson National Historic Park Campground

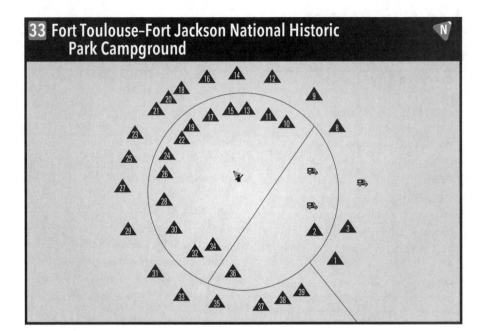

:: Getting There

From Wetumpka take AL 231 South 1.1 miles. Turn right onto West Fort Toulouse Road and travel 2.5 miles to the park entrance. The registration office is on the left.

GPS COORDINATES N32° 30.388'   W86° 15.155'

34

Frank Jackson State Park

"One of the out-of-the-way, off-the-beaten-path parks that is the perfect setting for rest, relaxation, and natural beauty"

I've commented elsewhere in this book that Alabama is blessed with some amazing state parks that showcase the state's natural beauty. These usually are the larger resort parks where throngs of people tend to gather.

Then there are the outliers, those small, out-of-the-way, off-the-beaten-path parks that are the perfect setting for rest, relaxation, and natural beauty. One of those is Frank Jackson State Park.

The park has operated since 1970, when it was originally known as Lightwood Knot Creek State Park. The name came from the creek that feeds the lake. In the 1980s the state changed the name to Frank Jackson in honor of a state representative from Covington County, where the park is located.

Located in the town of Opp, Frank Jackson encompasses 2,050 acres of land with its centerpiece being Lake Frank Jackson, a 1,037-acre natural stream-fed lake. This is one of the better fishing lakes you'll find, and it hosts a large bass tournament every April. The state touts it as a "premier fishing destination." Anglers can wet their line and try their hands at catching white or black crappie, largemouth bass, channel catfish, or bluegill. An Alabama freshwater-fishing license is required. There are concrete boat ramps and plenty of places to fish from the shoreline.

It's not all fishing at Frank Jackson, though. The park also has about 3 miles of beautiful hiking trails, including a boardwalk and bridge route that takes hikers to an island in the lake. A short interpretive loop circles the island to explore the flora and fauna. Be sure to pick up the informational flier at the kiosk before beginning the hike. Oh, and don't be afraid of the strange "visitors" in October and November. That is when local residents, schools, and businesses line the trails with whimsical creations for the annual Scarecrows in the Park event.

It's here that I need to sing the praises of the Trail Masters, a group of volunteers who help make the park as beautiful as it is. They began as a group of local residents who believed that Frank Jackson State Park was an asset to the area and wanted to contribute to its success. They began by building a new hiking trail and now take on many park projects, including creating and maintaining interpretive signs, trail maintenance, and general beautification projects.

Another event that brings crowds is the annual Opp Fest. Held in late October, the gathering celebrates the fall and harvest

:: Ratings

BEAUTY: ★ ★ ★ ★
PRIVACY: ★ ★ ★ ★
SPACIOUSNESS: ★ ★ ★ ★
QUIET: ★ ★ ★ ★
SECURITY: ★ ★ ★ ★
CLEANLINESS: ★ ★ ★ ★

:: Key Information

ADDRESS: 100 Jerry Adams Dr., Opp, AL 36467

OPERATED BY: Alabama State Parks

CONTACT: 334-493-6988; alapark.com/frankjackson

OPEN: Year-round

SITES: 31

SITE AMENITIES: Gravel pad, picnic table, fire ring with grate, grill, water, power

ASSIGNMENT: First-come, first-serve

REGISTRATION: At office

FACILITIES: Flush toilets, hot showers, laundry, Wi-Fi, boat ramp, fishing

PARKING: At each site

FEE: Waterfront sites, Sunday–Thursday, $27 (nonwaterfront, $24); waterfront sites, Friday–Saturday, $30 (non-waterfront, $27)

ELEVATION: 282'

RESTRICTIONS:

■ **Pets:** On leash only

■ **Fires:** In fire ring only; use only deadfall

■ **Alcohol:** Prohibited

■ **Vehicles:** 2/site

■ **Other:** Quiet hours 10 p.m.–6 a.m.; 8 people/site

season and is presented by the Opp Cultural Arts Council. The weekend is filled with arts and crafts, food vendors, music, children's activities, and more. Contact the council at 334-493-4880 for more information.

Your visit may include a wide variety of animals, ranging from flocks of songbirds to squirrels, deer, and, yes, alligators. Remember, don't feed them! Alligators would much rather leave humans alone, but when they are being fed by humans, the rules change. One sign in Alabama national forests and state parks says it all: $10,000 FINE FOR MOLESTING ALLIGATORS. (So . . . someone did that once?)

While we're on the subject of reptiles, the town of Opp is the home of the annual Rattlesnake Rodeo. Held each spring, the rodeo is everything rattlesnake, including shows, demonstrations, and even races.

The weekend is also a major arts and crafts festival with music and entertainment and lots of food (yes, even rattlesnake meat). You can read more about the rodeo at **rattlesnakerodeo.com.**

As for camping, all of the sites are very nice with compact crushed gravel pads, power, water, a picnic table, and a fire ring with a grate. Needless to say, the best sites are on the banks of the lake, 1–23. And if you can't live without Internet, Wi-Fi access is available.

The bathhouse is very spacious and clean with three hot showers, all handicap-accessible. There is also a coin-operated laundry here.

The park also has excellent security. The front gate has keypad entry, and for after-hour emergencies, the park manager lives on-site.

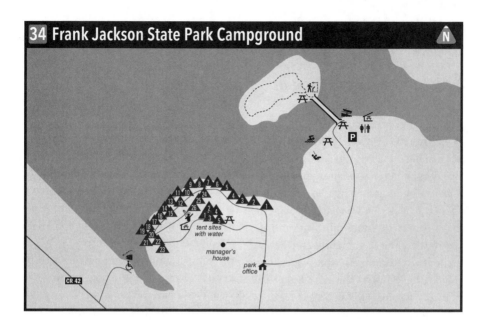

34 Frank Jackson State Park Campground

:: Getting There

From Opp take North Main Street 0.6 mile. Turn left onto West Jeffcoat Avenue/ Opine Road. Travel 1.1 miles and turn right onto Jerry Adams Drive. The park entrance is straight ahead.

GPS COORDINATES   N31° 17.839'   W86° 16.476'

35

Gunter Hill Campground

"A picture-postcard look at nature at its best in the South"

Just north of the state capital of Montgomery, two major rivers—the Tallapoosa and Coosa—converge to form the Alabama. The resultant river forms a much larger current that flows south through the central part of the state until it eventually merges with the Tombigbee and several other rivers to form the second-largest river delta in the country, the Mobile–Tensaw. Eventually, it spills into the Gulf of Mexico.

It's hard to believe that in the shadow of a major Southern city, along the muddy backwaters of this winding river, you will find a picture-postcard look at nature, but you do at this serene US Army Corps of Engineers campground.

Gunter Hill Campground is actually located on Catoma and Antioch Creeks, two of the many fingers of the river. Catoma is only one of two waterways in the state that flow to the north instead of south. *Catoma* is an American Indian word believed to be Muskogean in origin. The word loosely translates into "Tome water," the Tome being a subtribe of the Muskogean.

The campground has a natural, Southern laid-back feel to it, with thick stands of

:: Ratings

> **BEAUTY:** ★ ★ ★ ★
> **PRIVACY:** ★ ★ ★
> **SPACIOUSNESS:** ★ ★ ★
> **QUIET:** ★ ★ ★ ★
> **SECURITY:** ★ ★ ★ ★
> **CLEANLINESS:** ★ ★ ★ ★

hickory and pine trees. Gunter Hill has been called Spanish moss heaven. The growth is thick and forms beautiful and natural flowing light-green curtains. The campground abuts the Lowndes Wildlife Management Area, a protected state property. It's not uncommon to see some of that wildlife in the campgrounds, including deer and turkeys. I've heard that wild hogs are also in the vicinity but haven't seen any.

These backwaters provide fishing opportunities for anglers, the main catches being crappie, bass, and catfish. The campground has a boat ramp, and the creeks are also great paddling waters. The creeks offer plenty of sloughs and inlets to explore, which also serve as great places to watch some of the waterfowl, such as wood ducks and ospreys, that call these waters home.

You would think that the campground, being so close to the state capital, would overflow with visitors. In the summer it does get a bit crowded, mainly with day-trippers, but overall the campground is quiet and peaceful, with most of the campsites taking full advantage of the shade of those hickory trees. The loudest noise you will hear is the occasional jet from nearby Maxwell-Gunter Air Force Base, but those are few and far between and won't disturb your tranquility.

The campground has two loops, each named for the creeks on which they are located. The Antioch Loop includes sites 1–77 and the Catoma Loop has sites 78–146. Campsites are rather close together. You lose a little in privacy and quiet, but it's not a big

:: Key Information

ADDRESS: 561 Booth Rd., Montgomery, AL 36108

OPERATED BY: US Army Corps of Engineers

CONTACT: 334-872-9554; reservations 877-444-6777; tinyurl.com/gunterhill

OPEN: Year-round

SITES: 146

SITE AMENITIES: Grass or gravel pads, picnic table, fire ring, grill, lantern post, water, power

ASSIGNMENT: First-come, first-serve or by reservation

REGISTRATION: At entry gate or by reservation

FACILITIES: Flush toilets, hot showers, laundry, playground, basketball court, boat ramp, creek swimming, fishing

PARKING: At each site

FEE: Loop A, $20; Loop B, $22

ELEVATION: 356'

RESTRICTIONS:

■ **Pets:** On leash only; not allowed in beach areas, playgrounds, or restrooms

■ **Fires:** In fire ring or grill only; use only deadfall

■ **Alcohol:** Prohibited

■ **Vehicles:** 3/site

■ **Other:** Quiet hours 10 p.m.–6 a.m.; 8 people/site; must obtain pass and display in windshield before entering

drawback and shouldn't aversely disrupt your weekend. Each site has standard Corps of Engineers design, sporting dirt or compact crushed gravel pads, water, electricity, a picnic table, a fire ring, grill, and a lantern post.

A good number of sites are near the water and have nice views and cool breezes. In Catoma those would be 4–7 and 30–32, the latter being by far the best. In Antioch waterfront sites are 80–83, 90–91, 93–95, 97–104, 111, 113–114, and 117. All are right along the creek.

The two bathhouses are both located in the Antioch Loop. They are a bit older but quite nice and clean, with four hot showers in each men's and women's side. A coin-operated laundry is also available there.

For the kids, there are two playgrounds, as well as a basketball court, available in the Antioch Loop. A small general store stocks a limited number of items that you might have forgotten.

And lest I forget, Gunter Hill has excellent security, as do all of the Corps of Engineers campgrounds, with a main park attendant's station at the entrance and gates locked after-hours, plus camp hosts living just inside the entrance.

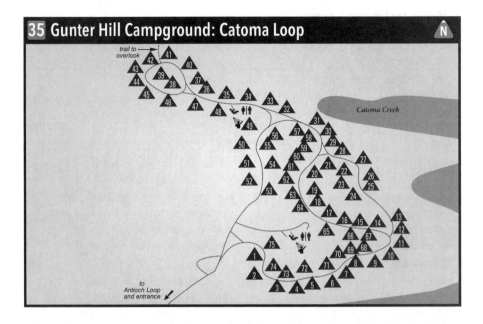

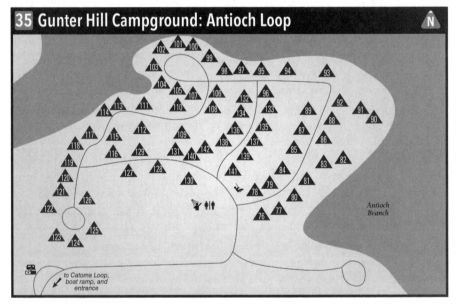

:: Getting There

From Montgomery take Maxwell Boulevard/Birmingham Highway 4 miles. Turn left onto West Boulevard. Travel 1.4 miles and turn right onto Old Selma Road. Travel 4.8 miles. Turn right onto Booth Road/County Road 7. Travel 0.5 mile. The entrance is on the right.

GPS COORDINATES   N31° 21.508'   W86° 27.300'

36

Hardridge Creek Campground

"What many call one of the finest campgrounds on the East Coast"

How does that old Alan Jackson song go? "Way down yonder on the Chattahoochee, never knew how much that muddy water meant to me." That sums up the locals' feeling about the river. Life along the muddy water seems to epitomize Southern life—laid-back and carefree, but full of fun. That fun comes from the multitude of recreational opportunities available along its banks, and the US Army Corps of Engineers accentuates those opportunities by providing what many call one of the finest campgrounds on the East Coast: Hardridge Creek Campground.

Hardridge is one of several Corps of Engineers campgrounds along the banks of Walter F. George Lake. The lake, also called Lake Eufaula, is the result of damming up the Chattahoochee River to produce hydroelectric power for the region, and the lake is one massive body of water. It has a surface area of 46,000 acres, has 640 miles of shoreline, and is 85 miles in length. Of course a body of water like this provides one big side benefit—recreation. Thousands of people come each year to fish, camp, and swim.

The US Army Corps of Engineers is responsible for much of the work on the nation's waterways. The Corps is divided into several divisions, which are subdivided into districts. The Mobile District supports projects such as the Walter F. George Lake and Hardridge Creek Campground in Alabama, but also similar projects in Mississippi, Georgia, and northwest Florida. It also maintains projects outside of the states in Guatemala, Honduras, El Salvador, Nicaragua, Columbia, Ecuador, Peru, and Bolivia.

Closer to home, back at Walter F. George Lake, the top activity is fishing. Anglers can cast a line for crappie, bream, several species of catfish, and, of course, bass, including largemouth and spotted. Hey, this is the Bass Fishing Capital of the World after all.

While you are at Hardridge Creek, I suggest that you take the time to visit the nearby town of Eufaula. It is steeped with history from before the Civil War to the present. One of the best times to visit is in late March during the Eufaula Pilgrimage, when the town provides a sampling of all of its rich history. Over three days, beautiful antebellum homes are open for tours. Many date to 1850 and are on the National Register

:: Ratings

BEAUTY: ★ ★ ★ ★
PRIVACY: ★ ★ ★ ★
SPACIOUSNESS: ★ ★ ★ ★
QUIET: ★ ★ ★ ★
SECURITY: ★ ★ ★ ★
CLEANLINESS: ★ ★ ★ ★

:: Key Information

ADDRESS: 592 U.S. Government Rd., Abbeville, AL 36310

OPERATED BY: US Army Corps of Engineers

CONTACT: 334-585-5945; reservations 877-444-6777; tinyurl.com/hardridge

OPEN: March–October

SITES: 77

SITE AMENITIES: Gravel pad, picnic table, prep table, fire ring, grill, lantern post, water, power

ASSIGNMENT: First-come, first-serve or by reservation (no reservations for sites 37–57)

REGISTRATION: At entry gate or by reservation

FACILITIES: Flush toilets, hot showers, laundry, playground, river swimming, fishing

PARKING: At each site; additional parking along the campground road at the Bayshore Loop

FEE: $20

ELEVATION: 238'

RESTRICTIONS:

■ **Pets:** On leash only; not allowed in beach areas, playgrounds, or restrooms

■ **Fires:** In fire ring or grill only; use only deadfall

■ **Alcohol:** Prohibited

■ **Vehicles:** 3/site

■ **Other:** Quiet hours 10 p.m.–6 a.m.; 8 people/site; reservations must be made 4 days in advance; 2-night minimum stay on weekends; 3-night minimum stay on holiday weekends; must obtain pass and display in windshield before entering

of Historical Places. One of the highlights is the candlelight home tour. You can also visit the First Presbyterian Church, which was built in 1869 in a Gothic style.

The weekend also features music, Civil War reenactments, carriage rides, plenty of food, and arts and crafts. Learn more at **eufaulapilgrimage.com.**

As with most Corps of Engineers campgrounds, Hardridge is clean and beautiful. The facility sports five loops, and many sites have excellent views of the lake or are located right on its banks. The best waterside sites are 1–12, 26–32, 38–41, 51–53, and 62–66. The absolute best lakeside sites are 42–45, which are situated on a narrow peninsula jutting out into the lake. It's simply beautiful.

The Bayshore Loop includes sites 1–22, Harbor Pass includes sites 23–36 (although site 36 lies outside of the loop along the main campground road), Pirates Cove has sites 37–47, Lake View has sites 48–54, and Shady Loop features sites 58–77. Each site has a compact crushed gravel pad, concrete parking area, water, electricity, a picnic table, a separate prep table, a grill, a fire ring, and a lantern post.

The campground has two recently renovated bathhouses, so they are modern and very clean. Each men's and women's side has two hot showers that are handicap-accessible and heated. A coin-operated laundry is also in each of the bathhouses.

As we've seen with all Corps of Engineers campgrounds, Hardridge has excellent security, with a park attendant station and locked gates after-hours, and the camp hosts live right next to the gates. They will give you a phone number in case of an after-hour emergency. (Speaking of camp hosts,

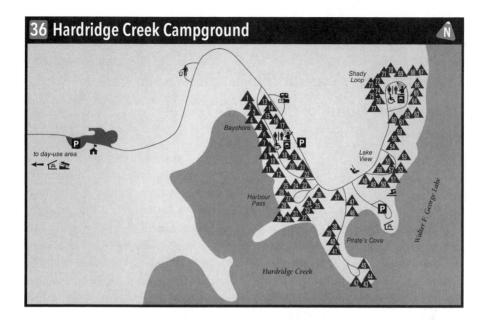

I have to compliment the ones I met while visiting Corps of Engineers campgrounds—always friendly and helpful.)

Please keep in mind that if you plan on reserving a site at Hardridge Creek Campground, you must make your reservation at least four days in advance. There is also a two-day minimum stay required on weekends and a three-day minimum stay required on holiday weekends.

:: Getting There

From Abbeville take AL 10 East 11.7 miles. Turn left onto County Road 237. Travel 0.6 mile, and turn left onto CR 46. Travel 0.2 mile and turn right onto CR 97. Travel 3.1 miles and turn right onto U.S. Government Road. The entrance is straight ahead in 0.2 mile.

GPS COORDINATES   N31° 38.609'   W85° 06.316'

37

Lakepoint Resort State Park

"You won't be wanting for things to do here in the
Bass Fishing Capital of the World."

Lake Eufaula, also known as Walter F. George Reservoir, covers 46,000 acres and was formed by the damming of the Chattahoochee River that borders Alabama and Georgia. The US Army Corps of Engineers also built a hydroelectric dam and lock that bears the same name. And while the river was dammed to provide navigation to the Gulf of Mexico and to provide power to the region, thousands of people each year flock to the area for the remarkable outdoor recreational opportunities it also provides. Smack dab in the middle of the lake is a fabulous Alabama state park resort, Lakepoint Resort.

The park itself covers 1,220 acres and offers a wide variety of activities. It's safe to say that you won't be wanting for things to do here. Of course it doesn't hurt that the park is in an area known as the Bass Fishing Capital of the World. On any given weekend you could find yourself in the midst of up to a dozen bass tournaments and heavy traffic on US 431 going into the park.

Other park amenities include two tennis courts—one located by the marina and the other in the campground between the Clark and Deer Court Loops. You'll also find seven hiking trails totaling about 5 miles, including a nice nature trail loop around the campground itself that follows the banks of the lake. Be sure to keep an eye out for a passing alligator in the water. Remember, don't bother it and it won't bother you—and keep your distance.

This is a resort park, which means Lakepoint has a championship caliber 18-hole golf course complete with a pro shop open seven days a week. And don't miss a swim in the lake. There is an excellent beach just east of Clark Loop. It is a short walk from the loop along the nature trail.

If you'd like something to eat besides the normal camp fare, the park boasts a wonderful restaurant that specializes in seafood. And if you want to stay at camp but forgot some essentials, the marina/store is well stocked.

Be sure not to spend all of your time at Lakepoint, though. The city of Eufaula has remarkable history, and the park is located next to the Eufaula National Wildlife Refuge with more than 11,000 acres of wetlands and upland habitats. You'll find hiking trails and observation platforms there.

Lakepoint Resort State Park has three camp loops: the Alabama, Barbour, and Clark. An additional loop, Deer Court, is RV only and where you will find the camp host at site 66.

:: Ratings

BEAUTY: ★ ★ ★ ★
PRIVACY: ★ ★ ★
SPACIOUSNESS: ★ ★ ★
QUIET: ★ ★ ★ ★
SECURITY: ★ ★ ★ ★
CLEANLINESS: ★ ★ ★ ★

:: Key Information

ADDRESS: 104 Lakepoint Dr., Eufaula, AL 36027

OPERATED BY: Alabama State Parks

CONTACT: 334-687-6026; alapark.com/lakepointresort

OPEN: Year-round

SITES: 127

SITE AMENITIES: Grass pad, picnic table, fire ring with grate, grill, water, power

ASSIGNMENT: First-come, first-serve or by reservation

REGISTRATION: At marina or by reservation

FACILITIES: Flush toilets, hot showers, laundry, tennis court, lake swimming, restaurant, camp store

PARKING: At each site

FEE: Clark Loop waterfront sites, Sunday–Thursday, $25 (Friday–Saturday, $28); Barbour and Clark Loops non-waterfront sites, Sunday–Thursday, $19 (Friday–Saturday, $22)

ELEVATION: 220'

RESTRICTIONS:

■ **Pets:** On leash only

■ **Fires:** In fire ring or grill only; use only deadfall or purchase at marina

■ **Alcohol:** Prohibited

■ **Vehicles:** 2/site

■ **Other:** Quiet hours 10 p.m.–6 a.m.; 8 people/site

The Alabama Loop is strictly tent camping. Sites mostly lack shade but are still very nice. No facilities are in this loop, but a short walk leads to the bathhouses in the Barbour Loop next door.

Barbour and Clark Loops are improved sites with all of the amenities—grass pad, power, water, grill, picnic table, and fire ring. The sites are relatively close together but not enough to disturb your peace and privacy. A heated bathhouse is located in each loop. Each has three hot, clean showers. The best sites are in the Clark Loop, where a dozen campsites sit directly on the lake under towering pines.

Don't be confused when you pull into the park to register. The registration office used to be at the campground itself but has been moved to the marina and store. So when you arrive, don't follow the sign that says CAMPGROUND and points to the left. Instead make a right turn and head to the marina. The campground is 1 mile away from the marina.

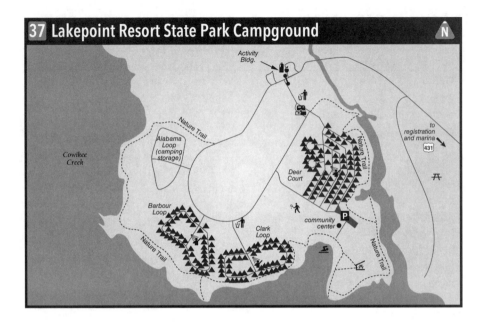

:: Getting There

From Eufaula take US 431/US 82 North 7.2 miles. Turn right onto Lakepoint Drive. Travel 0.2 mile and turn right. The marina where you register is to the left.

GPS COORDINATES   N31° 58.961'   W85° 06.566'

38

Millers Ferry Campground

"Plenty of opportunities for wildlife viewing and birding by canoe, kayak, or even the vestibule of your tent"

Millers Ferry Lock and Dam is another US Army Corps of Engineers project along the Alabama River that slows the flow of the river to make it navigable, control flooding, and generate power for the area. The resulting reservoir, Millers Ferry, or what is sometimes referred to as East Bank, covers more than 27 square miles, has more than 500 miles of shoreline, and creates an amazing network of wetlands and sloughs offering plenty of opportunities for wildlife viewing and birding by canoe, kayak, or even the vestibule of your tent.

Another beautiful US Army Corps of Engineers campground, Millers Ferry is located on a horseshoe bend of the river. Throughout the book I have discussed the Alabama and its importance to the region and the state, but recently the river has taken on another role as an important magnet for ecotourism, specifically as the backbone of the Alabama Scenic River Trail.

The trail is more than 600 miles long, using seven rivers and two creeks to run from Georgia to the Gulf of Mexico,

providing paddlers with an amazing view of the state and its natural beauty. The trail is the longest single blueway path in the country. The Alabama Scenic River Trail Association has partnered with many federal and state agencies to create the trail, including agreements for the use of campgrounds and locks along the route. Millers Ferry is one of those locks. Keep your eye out for paddlers while camping here and spend some time talking to them about their adventure. Most thru-trippers camp here along the way as they paddle the entire length of the river. You can learn more about the Alabama Scenic River Trail at **alabamascenicrivertrail.com.**

Another fantastic fishing river, the Alabama provides anglers an opportunity to land bass, crappie, bluegill, and catfish.

If you are looking for a night out in a waterfront campsite, then Millers Ferry is just for you, with all but a few of its 66 spots right on the Alabama River or pretty close. The only sites not directly on the banks are 26–28 and 41–60. The campground has set aside several sites that can be reserved, including 8–17, 22–25, 29–53, and 64–66. All others are first-come, first-serve.

Each site is equipped with a compact crushed gravel pad, water, electricity, a picnic table, a fire ring, a grill, and lantern posts. There is plenty of space between each site, so you are virtually guaranteed privacy and a quiet stay.

:: Ratings

BEAUTY: ★ ★ ★ ★
PRIVACY: ★ ★ ★ ★
SPACIOUSNESS: ★ ★ ★ ★
QUIET: ★ ★ ★ ★
SECURITY: ★ ★ ★ ★ ★
CLEANLINESS: ★ ★ ★ ★

:: Key Information

ADDRESS: 111 East Bank Park, Camden, AL 36726

OPERATED BY: US Army Corps of Engineers

CONTACT: 334-682-4191; reservations 877-444-6777; tinyurl.com/millersferry

OPEN: Year-round

SITES: 66

SITE AMENITIES: Gravel pads, picnic table, fire ring, grill, lantern post, water, power

ASSIGNMENT: First-come, first-serve or by reservation

REGISTRATION: At entry gate or by reservation

FACILITIES: Flush toilets, hot showers, laundry, playground, lake swimming, fishing, courtesy docks, all-purpose court

PARKING: At each site

FEE: Nonwaterfront sites, $18; waterfront sites, $20

ELEVATION: 92'

RESTRICTIONS:

■ **Pets:** On leash only; not allowed in swimming areas, playgrounds, or restrooms

■ **Fires:** In fire ring or grill only; use only deadfall

■ **Alcohol:** Prohibited

■ **Vehicles:** 3/site

■ **Other:** Quiet hours 10 p.m.–6 a.m.; 8 people/site; must obtain pass and display in windshield before entering; must hang lanterns from provided posts

The campground has 11 courtesy docks sprinkled along the banks of the river for you to tie up your boat, canoe, or kayak; better yet, just sit and watch the wildlife, birds, and river traffic from the dock. It's the perfect setting to watch the sun rise and watch a light fog roll down the river while you partake in a hot cup of coffee or tea. For fishermen, the campground also has a single cement boat launch between sites 17 and 18.

You'll find a diverse wildlife population living in the area. From your campsite you may catch a glimpse of a bald eagle or red-tailed hawk soaring high in the sky, hear the haunting hoots of a number of owls, or be lulled to sleep by a chorus of frog song. Frequently you will see beavers swimming in the backwaters, or glimpse white-tailed deer or wild turkeys cautiously moving through camp.

There are two bathhouses here, both exceptionally clean with two hot showers in each men's and women's side that are handicap-accessible. Both facilities also have coin-operated laundries. An extra restroom is located behind sites 58 and 59.

The campground has two very nice playgrounds. One is located just past the entrance gate across from sites 28 and 29, and the other is near the bathhouse next to site 45. And Millers Ferry has what is called an all-purpose court, suitable for volleyball, basketball, and even horseshoes (equipment is kept at the park attendant's station at the entrance).

With a gate locked after-hours and the park attendants or camp hosts living near the attendant station at the entrance, Millers Ferry has excellent security.

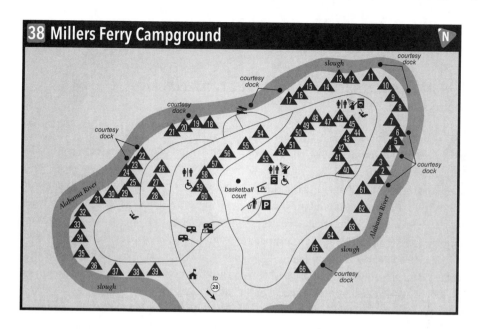

:: Getting There

From Camden take AL 28 West 10.7 miles. Turn right onto East Bank Road. Travel 0.2 mile to the entrance.

GPS COORDINATES   N33° 27.644'   W85° 52.489'

39

Open Pond Recreation Area

"Open Pond is spacious with guaranteed privacy."

Alabama is blessed with five national forests. The southernmost is Conecuh National Forest, an 83,000-acre longleaf-pine woodland on the Alabama–Florida state line.

Within the forest boundaries is the 450-acre Open Pond Recreation Area. Its 65 improved and 10 primitive sites are arranged in four loops. Sites are nicely separated and staggered for spaciousness and privacy.

Loops A and B are primitive sites. Loop A has 10 units that offer a good view of the pond wherever you pitch camp. The area has hard-packed pads, picnic tables, fire rings, and lantern posts. Loop B is a wide-open area for larger groups, such as Boy Scout troops. The only amenity is one fire ring in the field.

If you are looking for something a bit less rustic, then set up camp in loops C or D. Both feature fire rings, picnic tables, lantern posts, water spigots, and electricity at each site. Some have cement pads for RVs, but most are packed gravel or dirt. For a pond-side camp, arrive early for units on the south side of both loops. The friendly camp hosts, found at sites C26 or D21, have plenty of information. Bathhouses are very clean with flush toilets and hot showers. One is located at the far end of

loop D, one between loops C and D, one in Loop C, and one between loops A and C.

Remember, the recreation area can get crowded in early or late summer, but most of the time that isn't a problem. There is no campground gate, so you can arrive at your convenience; but the US Forest Service asks that you pay for your campsite at the entrance kiosk no later than 30 minutes after your arrival.

Open Pond is a beautiful campground that provides the perfect base camp from which to explore the wonders of this longleaf forest. To the north you can take a short drive up AL 137 to the Conecuh Trail's north trailhead and hike a short 0.5 mile to visit cypress-lined Nellie Pond. In the spring after the sun sets you will be treated to a frog chorus. The concert reverberates throughout the pine forest. The trail is lined with reflective white blazes to make it easy to hike at night.

To the south, several trails make their way around Ditch, Alligator, and Bucks Ponds, where you'll see a tremendous number of waterfowl and maybe an alligator or the endangered red-cockaded woodpecker. Then follow that up with a stroll down the Five Runs Loop Trail, a tranquil walk alongside its namesake creek, which is a wide feeder of the Yellow River. The trail also takes you to Blue Spring, which is exactly as named—a clear, deep-blue spring.

Fishing for bass and bream is allowed in all of the ponds either from their banks or some nice piers. (If you bring a boat, it can't be gas-powered.)

:: Ratings

BEAUTY: ★ ★ ★ ★
PRIVACY: ★ ★ ★ ★
SPACIOUSNESS: ★ ★ ★ ★
QUIET: ★ ★ ★ ★
SECURITY: ★ ★ ★
CLEANLINESS: ★ ★ ★ ★

:: Key Information

ADDRESS: 24481 AL 55, Andalusia, AL 36420

OPERATED BY: US Forest Service

CONTACT: 334-222-2555; tinyurl.com/openpond

OPEN: Year-round

SITES: 65 improved, 10 primitive

SITE AMENITIES: Improved–picnic table, fire pit, grill, lantern post, water spigot, power; Primitive–none

ASSIGNMENT: First-come, first-serve

REGISTRATION: Self pay at entrance

FACILITIES: Flush toilets, hot showers, playground

PARKING: At each site

FEE: Improved, $12; primitive, $6

ELEVATION: 266'

RESTRICTIONS:
- **Pets:** On leash only
- **Fires:** In fire pit only
- **Alcohol:** Prohibited
- **Vehicles:** 2/site
- **Other:** No swimming due to alligators

And if you have a telescope or binoculars, bring them along. Conecuh is one of the darkest forests you'll visit, and along the banks of the pond, stargazing is a premium.

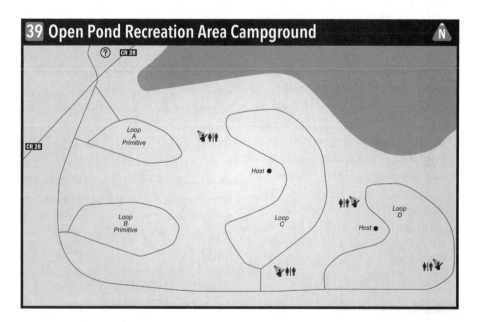

39 Open Pond Recreation Area Campground

:: Getting There

From Andalusia take US 29 South 11.2 miles. Turn left on AL 137. Travel 5.4 miles and turn left onto County Road 24. In 0.3 mile turn right onto CR 28. Follow CR 28 1.1 mile to the pay station.

GPS COORDINATES N31° 05.554' W86° 32.695'

40

Prairie Creek Campground

"Waterfront campsites, lake breezes, and Spanish moss–laden trees all add up to one splendid campout."

I am in awe of the beauty, cleanliness, and amenities at all of the US Army Corps of Engineers campgrounds in the state, but Prairie Creek has to top them all. The waterfront campsites, lake breezes, and Spanish moss–laden trees all add up to one splendid campout.

Prairie Creek is located on the banks of its namesake creek, a feeder of the Alabama River. The famed waterway begins its journey just north of Montgomery at the confluence of the Coosa and Tallapoosa Rivers. By the time it reaches Montgomery, the Alabama River is a deep, navigable watercourse, thanks to several dams established downstream by the US Army Corps of Engineers. These dams provide power to the region, as well as flood control and, our favorite byproduct, recreational activities such as the camping you will find here. This section of the river is part of Bob Woodruff Lake, which most locals call Jones Bluff Reservoir, created by the Robert Henry Lock and Dam.

This region of Alabama is rich in history, and a short 8-mile drive east of the

:: Ratings

BEAUTY: ★ ★ ★ ★ ★
PRIVACY: ★ ★ ★ ★
SPACIOUSNESS: ★ ★ ★ ★
QUIET: ★ ★ ★ ★
SECURITY: ★ ★ ★ ★ ★
CLEANLINESS: ★ ★ ★ ★

campground on County Road 29, you can experience a piece of that history at Holy Ground Battlefield Park.

The park is maintained by the Corps of Engineers and was a base for the Red Stick tribe of the Creek people during the Creek Indian War of 1813. It is here that American troops and allied Choctaws fought the Creeks led by William Weatherford. When the smoke cleared, 21 Creeks were killed and the rest were forced to retreat into the Alabama River. Weatherford, not wanting to be taken prisoner or worse, rode his gray horse, Arrow, off the edge of a 12-foot bluff and escaped by swimming to the opposite shore. You can learn more about the park by calling 334-875-6247.

As I said, Prairie Creek Campground is yet another beautiful, picturesque campground with Spanish moss–adorned hardwoods mixed with towering pines and some unbeatable waterfront campsites. The campground has two loops. Eagles Roost, on the banks of the creek, features sites 1–23, while Beaver Point has sites 24–62 and is located where the creek and river merge. All but a handful are either waterfront or pretty darn close, and all sites, both tent only and mixed use, are improved with compact crushed gravel pads, water, electricity, a picnic table, a fire ring, a grill, and a lantern post.

The Corps of Engineers was really looking after the tent camper on this one. Tent-only sites, if you can grab one, are 56–67 in

:: Key Information

ADDRESS: 582 Prairie Creek Rd., Lowndesboro, AL 36752	fish-cleaning station, courtesy docks
OPERATED BY: US Army Corps of Engineers	**PARKING:** At each site; Beaver Point Loop parking at end of loop (walk in to site)
CONTACT: 334-418-4919; reservations 877-444-6777; tinyurl.com/prairiecreek	**FEE:** $16
OPEN: Year-round	**ELEVATION:** 148'
SITES: 62	**RESTRICTIONS:**
SITE AMENITIES: Gravel pads, picnic table, fire ring, grill, lantern post, water, power	■ **Pets:** On leash only; not allowed in beach areas, playgrounds, or restrooms
ASSIGNMENT: First-come, first-serve or by reservation	■ **Fires:** In fire ring or grill only; use only deadfall
REGISTRATION: At entry gate or by reservation	■ **Alcohol:** Prohibited
	■ **Vehicles:** 3/site
FACILITIES: Flush toilets, hot showers, laundry, playground, fishing,	■ **Other:** Quiet hours 10 p.m.–7 a.m.; 8 people/site; must obtain pass and display in windshield before entering

the Beaver Point Loop. They are located on a peninsula jutting out into the river where Prairie Creek and the Alabama River meet. The cool lake breezes are wonderful and the views remarkable both at the campsites and at an overlook at the tip of the peninsula. Parking for tent-only sites is in a circular drive at the northern end of the campground road between sites 39 and 40. It is only a short walk to any of these sites.

Speaking of overlooks, another one, with a good view of the busy Alabama River, is located to the west and between sites 48 and 49.

As with several Corps of Engineers campgrounds along the Alabama River, Prairie Creek has eight courtesy docks as well as a cement boat ramp for boaters to use. Fishing is excellent along the banks or by boat. Largemouth and spotted bass as well as bream and crappie are only a few of the catches awaiting you. The campground has a convenient fish-cleaning station with running water.

Two playgrounds, one in each loop—as well as an all-purpose court that can be used for basketball or volleyball—entertain kids.

Prairie Creek has two bathhouses. These facilities are older but clean, with two hot showers in each men's and women's side. They are handicap-accessible and have coin-operated laundries.

Excellent security at the campground consists of gates locked after-hours and camp hosts living right next to them for your convenience.

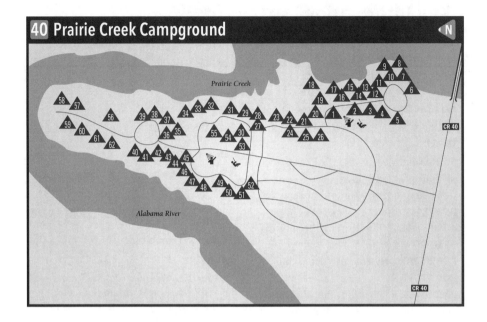

:: Getting There

From Lowndesboro take US 80 West 12.5 miles. Turn right onto Benton Road and travel 2.7 miles. Turn left onto County Road 40/Jones Bluff Road. Travel 1 mile and turn left onto Prairie Creek Road (this is a gravel road for the first 0.3 mile). The entrance gate is 0.5 mile ahead.

GPS COORDINATES   N32° 20.055'   W86° 46.204'

41

Six Mile Creek Campground

"Sounds of nature engulf you."

Look at the Alabama state seal and you can't help but notice the intricate web of rivers flowing through the state. One of the main waterways bisecting the state on that emblem is the Alabama River. Along this quintessential Southern river near the town of Selma is one of the scenic and peaceful US Army Corps of Engineers campgrounds that dot the muddy river's banks, Six Mile Creek.

The Alabama courses through the center of the state, flowing generally east to west before dipping south to meet up with the Tombigbee and its final journey to Mobile and the Gulf of Mexico. Several dams help make the river wide and navigable for commercial traffic. The second one from Montgomery, the Robert F. Henry Lock and Dam, forms the reservoir fed by Six Mile Creek. Dannelly Reservoir covers about 27 square miles with more than 500 miles of shoreline. Needless to say this means excellent fishing, with bass, crappie, bluegill, and catfish topping the list of catches.

The campground is located on the outskirts of Selma, a town steeped with history. Selma is most noted as being an epicenter of the civil rights movement in the 1960s.

:: Ratings

BEAUTY: ★ ★ ★ ★
PRIVACY: ★ ★ ★
SPACIOUSNESS: ★ ★ ★
QUIET: ★ ★ ★ ★
SECURITY: ★ ★ ★ ★ ★
CLEANLINESS: ★ ★ ★ ★

When in the area, be sure to take the time to visit the town and remember the fight for freedom and equality.

A few of the places you should take the time to visit include the Brown Chapel AME Church at 410 Martin Luther King Jr. Street. The church was the starting point for the famous Selma to Montgomery march. There were actually two marches. The first came on Sunday, March 7, 1965, when 600 protestors began the walk to the state's capital. They were met on the Edmund Pettus Bridge at the edge of town by state troopers; in what has become known as Bloody Sunday, the protestors were covered in tear gas and pummeled with billy clubs and bullwhips.

After hearing about what had occurred in Selma, thousands of people from across America flocked to the small town, and they began the walk anew, arriving at the state capital five days later. Five months later, President Lyndon Johnson signed the Voting Rights Act into law.

Also be sure to visit the Old Depot Museum at 4 Martin Luther King Jr. Street for a glimpse at the town's history from the Civil War to the 1960s. Learn more by calling 334-874-2197.

Six Mile Creek is a very peaceful campground, with the exception of weekends, when the area hosts one of the many bass tournaments. But generally the sounds of nature engulf you here, and with that comes the chance to spot wildlife, such as white-tailed deer, wild turkeys, raccoons, and possibly alligators. Remember, and I can't stress

:: Key Information

ADDRESS: 6485 County Road 77, Selma, AL 36701	**FACILITIES:** Flush toilets, hot showers, laundry, playground, fishing
OPERATED BY: US Army Corps of Engineers	**PARKING:** At each site
CONTACT: 334-872-9554; reservations 877-444-6777; tinyurl.com/sixmile	**FEE:** $16
	ELEVATION: 133'
OPEN: Year-round	**RESTRICTIONS:**
SITES: 31	■ **Pets:** On leash only; not allowed in beach areas, playgrounds, or restrooms
SITE AMENITIES: Gravel pads, picnic table, fire ring, grill, lantern post, water, power	■ **Fires:** In fire ring or grill only; use only deadfall
	■ **Alcohol:** Prohibited
ASSIGNMENT: First-come, first-serve or by reservation	■ **Vehicles:** 3/site
REGISTRATION: At entry gate or by reservation	■ **Other:** Quiet hours 10 p.m.–7 a.m.; 8 people/site; must obtain pass and display in windshield before entering

it enough, do not feed the gators. They are naturally afraid of humans, but feeding them changes the rules. And let me tell you, the gators do grow big in these parts. A state record alligator was caught in the area in 2011; it was more than 14 feet long and weighed in at 838 pounds!

All campsites have compact crushed gravel pads, water, electricity, a picnic table, a lantern post, a fire ring, and its own trash cans. The 31 sites are a bit close together but still have ample privacy. Sites 1–14 are in the Oak Valley Loop, and 15–31 are in Pine Bluff. In the Oak Valley Loop all but sites 1–3 are waterfront along the Six Mile Creek. In the Pine Bluff Loop, all but 15–17 and 22, 25, and 26 are located on the Alabama River.

The kids will enjoy the two playgrounds, one near the main entrance and one just before the Oak Valley Loop.

Individual restrooms are located just past the entrance and in the Oak Valley Loop. There is one bathhouse at the entrance to the Pine Bluff Loop. It's small, but considering the size of the campground and the number of visitors, it is more than adequate. The bathhouse has two hot showers and is handicap-accessible, but it is not heated.

Security is the same as at all Corps of Engineers facilities, with a main entrance office at the gate and entry gates that are locked after-hours. The camp hosts, who live next to the entrance, are very friendly and informative.

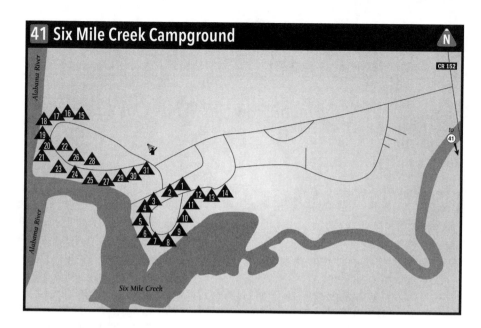

:: Getting There

From Selma take AL 8 0.6 mile. Turn right onto Kings Bend Road and travel 1.7 miles until the road becomes County Road 77. Travel another 0.6 mile. The entrance is on the right.

GPS COORDINATES   N32° 19.744'   W87° 00.609'

42

White Oak Creek Campground

"Fishing is one of the main draws; at White Oak Creek it is exceptional."

The Chattahoochee River, which borders Alabama and Georgia, begins its journey to the Gulf of Mexico in the Blue Ridge Mountains of north Georgia. There, several smaller streams merge, eventually becoming a wide, navigable river thanks to several dams and locks along its 436-mile-long journey to the sea. The river offers many beautiful places to camp, including this US Army Corps of Engineers property, White Oak Creek Campground.

White Oak is named for the creek inlet of the 46,000-acre Walter F. George Lake, created by a hydroelectric dam of the same name. The facility is located a mere 8 miles south of the town of Eufaula. *Eufaula* is an American Indian word, Muskogean in origin. Originally spelled *Yufala*, the word translates to "they separated here and went to the other place," an appropriate phrase considering the turbulent history of the area.

This area was the home of the Creek people for centuries when in 1831 General William Irwinton built a 31,000-acre estate along the river that included a steamboat wharf designed to take advantage of river-boat traffic. The problem was that, although Irwinton's home was on legally settled white land, the wharf was on Creek land.

In 1832 some of the Creek Nation signed a treaty that required the Creeks to move west of the Mississippi River, but many more did not agree to those terms and continued to live in the region, including on the land where Irwinton's wharf was located.

President Andrew Jackson sent Francis Scott Key to investigate claims of fraud being perpetrated against the Creeks still living here. The situation came to a head in 1836 when the Yuchi Branch of the Creek Nation, tired of the treatment and loss of their land, rose against the whites in what became known as the Creek War of 1836. Irwinton's home was used as one of the bases for federal troops as they forcibly removed the tribe from the land; that removal is now known as the Trail of Tears.

More than a century later, the damming of the river by the Corps of Engineers has provided some remarkable recreational opportunities for visitors to the area. As is the case all along the Chattahoochee River, fishing is one of the main draws; at White Oak Creek it is exceptional, with largemouth bass, bigmouth buffalo, bream, and bluegill being the main catches. There is also excellent fly-fishing along the area's many creeks

:: Ratings

BEAUTY: ★ ★ ★ ★
PRIVACY: ★ ★ ★ ★
SPACIOUSNESS: ★ ★ ★ ★
QUIET: ★ ★ ★ ★
SECURITY: ★ ★ ★ ★
CLEANLINESS: ★ ★ ★ ★

:: Key Information

ADDRESS: 395 AL 95, Eufaula, AL

OPERATED BY: US Army Corps of Engineers

CONTACT: 334-687-3101; reservations 877-444-6777; tinyurl.com/whiteoakcreek

OPEN: Year-round

SITES: 130

SITE AMENITIES: Gravel pad, picnic table, prep table, fire ring, grill, lantern post, water, power

ASSIGNMENT: First-come, first-serve or by reservation

REGISTRATION: At entry gate or by reservation

FACILITIES: Flush toilets, hot showers, laundry, playground, river swimming, fishing

PARKING: At each site; additional parking along the campground road at the Bayshore Loop

FEE: $22

ELEVATION: 255'

RESTRICTIONS:

■ **Pets:** On leash only; not allowed in beach areas, playgrounds, or restrooms

■ **Fires:** In fire ring or grill only; use only deadfall

■ **Alcohol:** Prohibited

■ **Vehicles:** 3/site

■ **Other:** Quiet hours 10 p.m.–6 a.m.; 8 people/site; 2-night minimum stay on weekends; 3-night minimum stay on holiday weekends; reservations must be made 4 days in advance; gate closed 10 p.m.–7 a.m.; must obtain pass and display in windshield before entering

and streams. Remember your Alabama freshwater-fishing license. The campground caters to fishermen with two cement boat ramps and a fish-cleaning station next to the park attendant's station.

The campground has four loops. Mallard Point hosts sites 1–29, Oakwood consists of sites 30–59, Creek View has sites 60–100, and River Chase features sites 60–130. All are open to walk-ins, although spots in Oakwood and Creek View Loops can be reserved. Reservations must be made four days in advance of your visit. Also remember that a two-night minimum reservation is required on weekends, and a three-night minimum is enforced on holiday weekends.

Every site includes a compact crushed gravel pad, power, water, a picnic table, a grill, a fire ring, a lantern post, and something rather unique—a table for kitchen work or prepping the fish you caught for dinner.

For water views sites 1–16 and 21, 22, and 24 in the Mallard Point Loop; 30–51 in the Oakwood Loop; and all but 75, 76, 79, 81, 84, 85, 89, 97, and 98 of the Creek View Loop provide excellent, unobstructed views of White Oak Creek. Sites 114–123 of River Chase offer the best views of Walter F. George Lake and the busy maritime traffic along its waters.

Each loop has its own bathhouse and, as with all Corps campgrounds along the river, are extremely clean. Each men's and women's side has two hot showers and is handicap-accessible, although the facilities are not heated. A nice touch is that while most campgrounds have only one laundry,

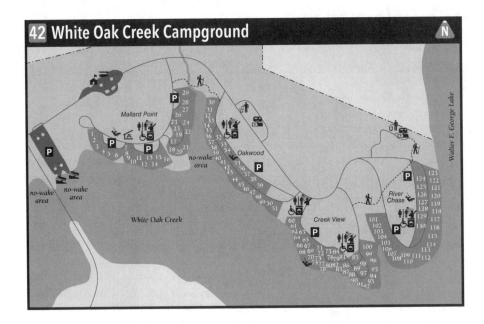

each bathhouse at White Oak has its own coin-operated laundry.

Another bonus is that all four loops have their own playgrounds. The best one is in the Creek View Loop next to site 70, which is right on a sandy beach overlooking the creek.

The campground has excellent gated security, and the park attendant lives right next to the entrance.

:: Getting There

From Eufaula take South Eufaula Avenue 6.9 miles. Turn left onto AL 95 South and travel 0.9 mile. The entrance is on the left.

GPS COORDINATES N31° 46.655' W85° 09.206'

Gulf Region

Blakeley Historic State Park

"A quiet getaway in the woods with plenty of beauty and history but without the tourist trappings"

If you're looking for a quiet getaway in the woods with plenty of beauty and history but without the tourist trappings of larger campgrounds, then Blakeley Historic State Park is just for you.

Blakeley is located on the banks of the second-largest river delta in the country, the Mobile–Tensaw River Delta. The delta covers more than 20,000 acres (about 30 miles by 20 miles in area) and has been described as an environmental showplace with more than 500 species of plants, 300 species of birds, 124 species of fish, 69 species of reptiles . . . well, you get the idea.

The delta is formed by the confluence of five rivers funneling water from several Southeastern states to Mobile Bay and eventually into the Gulf of Mexico.

A visit to Blakeley is highlighted by a beautiful walk on an elevated boardwalk along the shores of the delta, as well as by treks through the surrounding forest on more than 15 miles of trail.

Blakeley is not only a natural wonder but is also steeped in history. The park is located on the site of the old town of Blakeley. In

the early 1800s the town rivaled its cross-bay counterpart, Mobile, as one of the busiest port cities in the country. A yellow fever epidemic in the mid-1800s put an end to that, wiping out much of the population, with the survivors fleeing to other areas.

The town fell into ruin until it was repopulated by the Confederate Army during the Civil War and was a key defense for Mobile. On April 9, 1865, the North and South fought it out on these grounds in what would be the last major battle of the conflict. As the battle waged on, General Robert E. Lee surrendered his troops to General Ulysses S. Grant at Appomattox Court House in Virginia, thus effectively ending the war. Many of the hiking trails at Blakeley take visitors to remnants of the battle, including some of the best-preserved breastworks and redoubts in the country.

With easy access to the delta, Blakeley offers an excellent landing for launching a canoe or kayak. The park does not rent them here, so bring your own or rent them at any number of local outfitters. Be warned, however, that the delta is not for beginner paddlers. It's very easy to get lost in the backwaters and bayous, so be sure to get expert advice before heading out.

If you're not into paddling, then take a cruise up the delta on the park's own pontoon boat. Call ahead to check on hours of operation and for current prices.

If you're a first-time visitor or even if it's simply been awhile since you have been

:: Ratings

BEAUTY: ★ ★ ★ ★
PRIVACY: ★ ★ ★ ★
SPACIOUSNESS: ★ ★ ★
QUIET: ★ ★ ★ ★
SECURITY: ★ ★ ★ ★
CLEANLINESS: ★ ★ ★ ★

:: Key Information

ADDRESS: 34745 AL 225, Fort, AL 36527	**FACILITIES:** Flush toilets, hot showers
	PARKING: At each site
OPERATED BY: Alabama Historic Commission	**FEE:** Adults, $6/night; children (ages 6-12), $4/night
CONTACT: 251-626-0798; blakeleypark.com	**ELEVATION:** 211'
OPEN: Year-round	**RESTRICTIONS:**
SITES: 28	■ **Pets:** On leash only
SITE AMENITIES: Picnic table, fire ring	■ **Fires:** In fire ring only; use only deadfall or purchase at office
ASSIGNMENT: First-come, first-serve or by reservation	■ **Alcohol:** Prohibited
	■ **Vehicles:** 2/site
REGISTRATION: Pay attendant at office or by reservation	■ **Other:** Quiet hours 10 p.m.–6 a.m.; 1 tent (4 adults, 4 children)/site

to Blakeley, you're in for a treat. The park recently renovated the campgrounds. Each campsite is tucked away neatly within the towering pines, oaks, and magnolia trees, and the sites are spaced far apart, so you are guaranteed a peaceful and private stay.

While Blakeley is a favorite camping site for large groups of Boy Scouts, there's no need to worry about them disturbing you. The group campground is far enough away that you won't even hear them.

Each site has a picnic table and fire ring with a grate for grilling and ample parking. The tent pads are natural earth and very level. Plus each site has its own trash can, so there's no excuse not to practice "leave no trace" principles.

Security is quite good, with a gated entrance and a camp host to help out after-hours. A big park improvement is a brand-new modern bathhouse, situated at the campground entrance. On the east side there are wide and spacious restrooms, and to the west are new hot showers. And the facility is heated.

A good time to visit is the first weekend of April, when the site comes alive with reenactors re-creating the famous Civil War battle. Another exciting time is the first weekend of October, when the site hosts the Blakeley Bluegrass Festival. Both weekends are very popular, so make camping reservations early.

One word of warning: Late spring brings yellow flies. These pesky biting bugs are ferocious and are usually found near swamps, ponds, and riverbanks in shaded, humid areas—which is a perfect description of where Blakeley is located. You may want to contact the office during this time before heading out to check on the yellow fly situation.

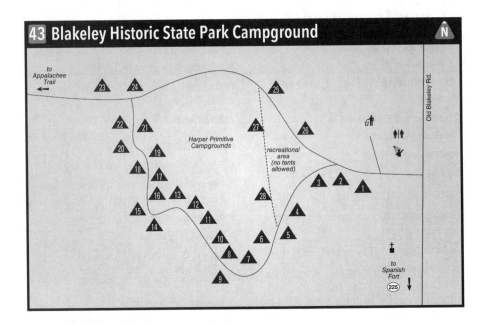

:: Getting There

From Spanish Fort take AL 225 North 5 miles. The entrance is on the left.

GPS COORDINATES   N30° 43.943'   W87° 53.974'

44

Chickasabogue Park

"This 1,100-acre park has something to keep even the most fidgety of youngsters occupied."

This is one family-friendly park. Operated by the Mobile County Parks and Recreation Department, this 1,100-acre park has something to keep even the most fidgety of youngsters occupied while providing plenty for adults, too.

Chickasabogue Park is located in the east-central part of Mobile County in a heavily populated area, but once you pass through the gates, you enter another world. It lives up to its mission to "provide a wide variety of outdoor activity while protecting the environment and preserving the diversity of plants and animals indigenous to the area."

And yes, wildlife abounds in this safe haven away from the maddening crowd. You may come across deer, foxes, raccoons, armadillos, and alligators during your visit. It goes without saying, but do not feed the alligators! They are naturally afraid of humans and would rather avoid you, but feeding them changes the game.

Chickasabogue has a long and storied history. American Indians lived on this site as early as 1500 B.C. Europeans made their first appearance in 1540 A.D. when Spanish explorer Hernando de Soto worked his way up from the Gulf of Mexico through what is now the state of Alabama.

The French made their first appearance in the area in 1711 but did not settle here until 1787, when Spanish Grandee Don Diego Miguel Alvarez received a grant to build a residence on the north bank of Chickasaw Creek.

Plenty of fun will be had by kids of all ages at Chickasabogue Park. And yes, that includes you, parents. Of course there are your standard campground activities, including fishing in Chickasaw Creek, which teems with bass, crappie, catfish, and pickerel (a freshwater-fishing license is required).

Speaking of the Chickasaw Creek, it is a great place to paddle. Bring your own canoe or rent one to float lazily down the beautiful stream. Its white sandy beaches welcome swimmers. Or if you like to hike or mountain bike, then take a trek over the park's 11 miles of trail.

An on-site museum traces regional history. It's located at the entrance of the park in the former Eight Mile AME Methodist Church building, which was built in 1879.

Oh, and did I mention that there is a Professional Disc Golf Association-sanctioned disc golf course here? Not to mention ball fields, basketball courts, and playgrounds.

:: Ratings

BEAUTY: ★ ★ ★
PRIVACY: ★ ★ ★
SPACIOUSNESS: ★ ★ ★
QUIET: ★ ★
SECURITY: ★ ★ ★ ★
CLEANLINESS: ★ ★ ★

:: Key Information

ADDRESS: 760 Aldock Rd.,
Eight Mile, AL 36613

OPERATED BY: Mobile County
Commission

CONTACT: 251-574-2267;
tinyurl.com/chickasaboguepark

OPEN: Year-round

SITES: 47

SITE AMENITIES: Picnic table, fire ring
with grill, water, power

ASSIGNMENT: First-come, first-serve

REGISTRATION: Pay attendant at office

FACILITIES: Flush toilets, hot showers,
laundry, trash cans, museum

PARKING: At each site

FEE: Improved (with power and water/

tents only/for 4 people), $10; improved
(with power and water/for 4 people),
$15; improved (with power, water, and
sewer/for 4 people), $18; primitive, $5
(for 2 people); add $2.50 for each addi-
tional person; add $5 for additional tent

ELEVATION: 28'

RESTRICTIONS:

■ **Pets:** On leash only

■ **Fires:** In fire ring only; use only deadfall

■ **Alcohol:** Prohibited

■ **Vehicles:** 2/site

■ **Other:** Quiet hours 8 p.m.–7 a.m.;
2 tents/site

After a busy day it's time to turn in, and the campsites at Chickasabogue Park are delightful. Each one is nestled under towering oaks, pines, and flowering dogwood trees. Ample spacing between sites keeps your privacy and maintains quiet.

You can either pitch your tent on a light compact gravel bed or the grassy areas next to each site. There is plenty of room for two vehicles in each site's pull-in or circular parking area.

Two clean bathhouses are located at the entrance to the south camp loop (sites 14–38) and the east camp loop (sites 1–13). A coin-operated laundry is also available and located next to the bathhouse at the south camp loop.

Chickasabogue Park has excellent security. The gate is locked after sunset, and security guards routinely patrol the campgrounds. They can assist if you need to enter or exit after-hours.

The only drawback to camping at Chickasabogue is the constant sound of cars rushing by on nearby I-65. It's not an obnoxious noise, simply in the background, but it's just enough to let you know that it's there.

An interesting possibility for camping, one that's outside the scope of this book, is the park's backcountry primitive sites. TOn the banks of Chickasaw Creek, they can be reached only by either hiking 15–20 minutes on a trail or by canoe.

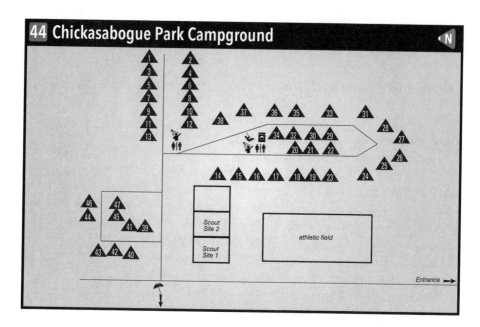

:: Getting There

From Eight Mile head northeast on South Shelton Beach Road 0.8 mile. Turn right onto North Whistler Street. Travel 0.8 mile. Turn left onto Aldock Road and travel 0.9 mile. The entrance is on the right.

GPS COORDINATES   N30° 46.742'   W88° 06.444'

45

Gulf State Park

"As close to resort lodging as you can get in a state park"

The **Alabama Gulf Coast** has seen its share of disasters over the past several years. In 2004, 2005, and 2006 the area was hit hard by a succession of hurricanes, including Ivan, Dennis, and Katrina. Ivan was by far the worst, scoring a direct hit on Gulf Shores with 130-mile-per-hour winds and a storm surge of 10–12 feet that forced water inland almost a mile.

Then in 2010 the *Deepwater Horizon* oil rig exploded, coating the coast from Louisiana to Florida with crude oil. Next, in 2011, a fire threatened the park, burning more than 400 acres of pine forest and wetlands.

But Alabama is resilient and the Gulf Coast has bounced back—big time! The beaches are pristine white again, and businesses are open and booming.

The Alabama Gulf Coast offers plenty of fun. The peninsula is the home of Bon Secour National Wildlife Refuge. Literally translated, the name means "safe haven," and it serves as the habitat for hundreds of species of rare wildlife and plants. You can explore these beautiful wetlands and beaches on more than 6 miles of trail.

Only 22 miles away to the west is Fort Morgan Historic State Park. During the Civil War, this stone garrison was one of the last bastions of the Confederacy and became famous for the conflict that was later called the Battle of Mobile Bay in which Union Admiral David Farragut reportedly uttered those famous words "Damn the torpedoes, full speed ahead!"

And of course, the Gulf Coast has miles of beautiful white beaches. In the heart of all of this you'll find Alabama's most popular state park, Gulf State Park. This is as close to resort lodging at a state park as you can get. It offers a campground boasting 15 miles of hiking trails, 496 campsites, tennis courts, a pool, a nature center, a playground, and a well-stocked, and I mean well-stocked, camp store.

The campgrounds are not only connected by the main camp road but also by hiking trails built by park staff and snowbirds (retirees coming down from the North to escape winter). And if you enjoy hiking or biking, check out the nearby Hugh S. Branyon Backcountry Trails, beautiful paved multiuse paths that wind their way through maritime wetlands lined with huge trees draped with Spanish moss.

Oh, and for the fishermen, the park boasts the largest gulf fishing pier at 1,540 feet. Don't forget your saltwater fishing license. And if you don't fish, it's still a beautiful 0.25-mile walk out into the gulf.

You can pitch your tent on light gravel or grass pads. Each site is improved with a

:: Ratings

BEAUTY: ★ ★ ★ ★
PRIVACY: ★ ★ ★
SPACIOUSNESS: ★ ★ ★
QUIET: ★ ★ ★ ★
SECURITY: ★ ★ ★ ★ ★
CLEANLINESS: ★ ★ ★ ★ ★

:: Key Information

ADDRESS: 22050 Campground Rd., Gulf Shores, AL 36542

OPERATED BY: Alabama State Parks

CONTACT: 251-948-7275; 800-252-7275; alapark.com/gulfstate

OPEN: Year-round

SITES: 496

SITE AMENITIES: Picnic table, grill, water, power

ASSIGNMENT: First-come, first-serve

REGISTRATION: Pay attendant at office or by reservation

FACILITIES: Flush toilets, hot showers, laundry, boat launch, tennis, pool, camp store

PARKING: At each site

FEE: Lakefront site on Gator Road or Live Oak nonwaterfront site (for 4 people), $34; Live Oak lakefront site or pull-through site across from lake, $37; lakefront pull-through site, $41; March–October, Friday–Saturday, $3 additional fee; add $5 for additional tent

ELEVATION: Sea level

RESTRICTIONS:

■ **Pets:** On 6-foot leash only

■ **Fires:** In grill only

■ **Alcohol:** Prohibited

■ **Vehicles:** 2/site

■ **Other:** Quiet hours 10 p.m.–6 a.m.; 1 tent (8 people)/site, extra tent for children allowed; 2-night minimum stay May–November, Friday–Saturday; 3-night minimum stay major holidays and special events; 14-day stay limit April–October

picnic table, a grill, water, and power. Fires are permitted only in grills, and after the recent fire, it's understandable that the rule is strictly enforced.

The bathhouses are modern and immaculate, and there are plenty, 11 altogether, to handle the crowds. In addition, a laundry is available at the camp store.

The best sites are 16–39 and 229–232, which are located along Middle Lake, a gorgeous freshwater lagoon where you can fish or just sit around and enjoy the view. Keep in mind that south Alabama has alligators, and they are prevalent in the park. Do not feed them! The reptiles are naturally afraid of humans, but feeding them changes the rules. Look from a distance and enjoy.

There is excellent security at the campground. It is gated with a large office for the park enforcement rangers, who provide 24-hour service and allow passage to and from the campground.

The only drawback to the campsites is their close proximity to one another. The tight quarters reduce privacy, but overall the sites are pleasant and fairly quiet.

So when is the best time to visit? Good question. The campsite bustles most any time of the year. Your best bet is to call ahead for reservations, although you may find that campsites have been booked several months in advance. Keep in mind that the winter is busy, too, as Northern retirees come down to escape the cold.

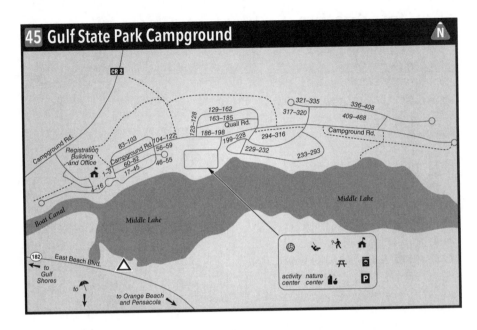

:: Getting There

At the intersection of US 59 and AL 180/West Beach Boulevard in Gulf Shores, head east on AL 180 2.2 miles. Turn left onto County Road 2/State Park Road 2 North. Travel 0.5 mile and turn right onto Campground Road. Travel 0.3 mile to the camp entrance.

GPS COORDINATES   N30° 15.587'   W87° 38.935'

46

Isaac Creek Campground

"Quiet beauty envelops you."

To be honest, Isaac Creek Campground was the first site that I visited while researching this book, and while I have been to many campgrounds across the state before, I had never been to a US Army Corps of Engineers site before. I'm sorry that I didn't visit them sooner, especially Isaac Creek.

This region along the Alabama River near the town of Monroeville is called the Red Hills, and it is here that the endangered Red Hills salamander lives. The campground lies nestled on a finger of land between the banks of the Alabama River and Isaac Creek, a wide waterway that feeds the river and lends its name to the campground. It's a beautiful example of what camping should be. Quiet beauty envelops you most days of the year, and even on those days where it gets a little more crowded, you will still find it idyllic.

The campground has 60 sites, all improved with power, water spigots, a picnic table, lantern post, and fire ring with attached grill. Each site has a cement drive for parking and a level, hard-packed gravel tent pad.

:: Ratings

BEAUTY: ★ ★ ★ ★
PRIVACY: ★ ★ ★ ★ ★
SPACIOUSNESS: ★ ★ ★ ★ ★
QUIET: ★ ★ ★ ★
SECURITY: ★ ★ ★ ★
CLEANLINESS: ★ ★ ★ ★

Some say that Isaac Creek is rustic. On the contrary, the amenities are top-notch. The two bathhouses within the camp loop are well kept and offer hot showers and laundry facilities. And three modern playgrounds plus a basketball court entertain the kid in each of us.

If you want a site with a view, then make your reservations early for sites 15–41. Those on the west side of the campground (15–31) are situated along Isaac Creek itself. You will find that all campsites offer ample room to ensure your privacy no matter how crowded the park. The creek is wide with a great Southern bayou feel. If you are a paddler, bring your boat. A courtesy dock is located between each of these sites.

The remaining waterfront sites face the Alabama River or Claiborne Lake, which is formed by the nearby Claiborne Lock and Dam. Built in 1971, the dam created this 60-mile-long lake that not only provides navigation for barges heading to the Gulf of Mexico but also offers plenty of recreational activities, including boating, fishing, and waterskiing.

Claiborne is the southernmost dam on the US Army Corps of Engineers' Alabama River lakes system. In all, three locks and dams make up this 245-mile waterway. The river is also part of one of the longest canoe trails in the country, the Alabama Scenic Rivers Trail.

A few hiking trails start near the campground. Among them is a moderate, 2.4-mile out-and-back walk up Haines Mountain.

:: Key Information

ADDRESS: 1226 Power House Rd., Camden, AL 36726

OPERATED BY: US Army Corps of Engineers

CONTACT: 334-682-4244; tinyurl.com/isaaccreek

OPEN: Year-round

SITES: 60

SITE AMENITIES: Picnic table, fire ring with grill, lantern post, water spigot, power

ASSIGNMENT: Some first-come, first-serve; mostly by reservation

REGISTRATION: National Recreation Reservation Service 877-444-6777 or pay attendant at gate

FACILITIES: Flush toilets, hot showers, laundry, playgrounds, basketball court, dock, museum

PARKING: At each site

FEE: Nonwaterfront sites, $18; waterfront sites, $20

ELEVATION: 92'

RESTRICTIONS:

■ **Pets:** On leash only

■ **Fires:** In grill or fire ring only

■ **Alcohol:** Prohibited

■ **Vehicles:** 3/site

■ **Other:** Quiet hours 10 p.m.–6 a.m.; gate closed 10 p.m.–7 a.m.; 8 people/site; limit 6 visitors/site (must leave by 9:30 p.m.); swimming is prohibited; 14-day stay limit

When hiked in the fall, the trail reminds many of the New England woods, as the leaves of Haines Mountain blaze with glorious color and, below, beaver dams create glistening ponds. At the summit you may meet up with the ghost of Nancy. The legend is a favorite tale told by park rangers. The story goes that Nancy once lived atop the mountain and remains there today waiting for the return of her husband from the Civil War.

During your stay, be sure to pay a visit to the Alabama River Museum. It's located just outside the campground entrance next to the dam. As you walk the museum halls, you will travel back in time to view ancient fossils, American Indian artifacts, and the river's steamboat era. A special treat comes the second week of March when the museum hosts the Alabama River Festival. It showcases the rich history of the region with food, music from the 1800s, and reenactors demonstrating life as it was along the river. The museum is open on Saturdays only, March–October, 9 a.m.–4 p.m. Admission is free.

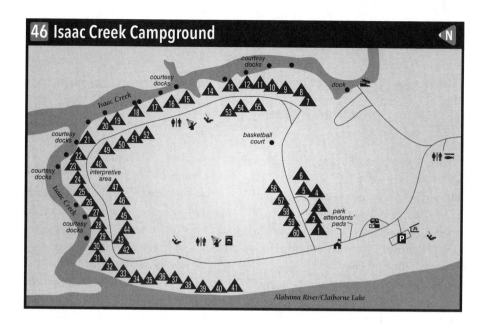

:: Getting There

From Monroeville take AL 41 North 9.2 miles. Turn left onto County Road 17. Travel 5 miles and turn left onto Finchburg Road. Travel 1.7 miles and turn left onto Lock and Dam Road. Follow the road 4 miles to the dam. Turn right onto Isaac Creek Road and travel 0.3 mile.

GPS COORDINATES   N31° 37.450'   W87° 33.010'

47

Little River State Forest

"What the park lacks in facilities, it more than makes up for with its recreation and beauty."

Little River State Forest is an out-of-the-way gem just north of Atmore. The Alabama Forestry Commission maintains this 2,100-acre woodlands, which is a typical Southern longleaf pine forest without the typical landscapes you will see elsewhere this close to the Gulf Coast.

The forest is divided almost right down the middle by AL 21. Meandering along the back roads on the west side, you will find the rare pitcher plant, a carnivorous oddity that thrives in seepage bogs like those found in pine forests along creek banks and riverbanks. Equally striking are the rock outcrops, something almost completely unheard of along Alabama's Gulf Coast. To the east of AL 21, you'll find the campground. As with most state parks in the region, the Civilian Conservation Corps (CCC) created this recreation area in 1935 and called it Little River State Park.

President Franklin Roosevelt created the CCC at the height of the Great Depression to give young men, generally ages 18–21, a job and to build an amazing infrastructure that helped lift the country out of economic turmoil. The men earned up to $30 a month, with $25 sent back to their parents. The work was backbreaking, but the craftsmanship was remarkable. A first-class example of their work can be seen on the park's Gazebo Trail, a 4-mile out-and-back that takes you to the trail's namesake gazebo. This is the original CCC structure, and its wooden framing and stonework stand as strong as they did 80 years ago.

The park itself has been through hard times, as well as a few name changes. In the mid-1970s it was renamed in honor of Atmore native and conservationist Claude D. Kelley. In 2004 and 2005, the area was hit by two major hurricanes, Ivan and Dennis, respectively. The park's infrastructure was severely damaged, and Alabama State Parks relinquished control to the Alabama Forestry Commission, which changed the park's name to Little River State Forest.

Recently, because of economic downturns, the commission was nearly forced to shut down the park, which would have been devastating to the hundreds of locals who flock here during the summer. Instead, Iron Men Outdoor Ministries, a nonprofit organization, took on park management, and today it is a thriving oasis for the residents of Escambia and Monroe Counties.

It is true that the campground has seen better days (it is more than 70 years old, after all), but Iron Men Outdoor Ministries is taking on the task of modernizing the facility.

:: Ratings

BEAUTY: ★ ★ ★ ★
PRIVACY: ★ ★ ★
SPACIOUSNESS: ★ ★
QUIET: ★ ★ ★
SECURITY: ★ ★ ★
CLEANLINESS: ★ ★ ★

:: Key Information

ADDRESS: 580 H. Kyle Rd., Atmore, AL 36502	**FACILITIES:** Flush toilets, hot showers, playground, swimming
OPERATED BY: Alabama Forestry Commission	**PARKING:** At each site
CONTACT: 251-862-2511; tinyurl.com/lrstateforest	**FEE:** Improved, $20; primitive, $10
	ELEVATION: 206'
OPEN: Year-round	
SITES: 12 improved, 20 primitive	**RESTRICTIONS:**
SITE AMENITIES: Improved–picnic table, grill, water, power; Primitive–picnic table, fire ring	■ **Pets:** On leash only
	■ **Fires:** In grill only
ASSIGNMENT: First-come, first-serve	■ **Alcohol:** Prohibited
REGISTRATION: At entrance gate or park office	■ **Vehicles:** 2/site
	■ **Other:** Quiet hours 10 p.m.–6 a.m.; 1 tent (4 people)/site

The campground itself is removed from the park's centerpiece 25-acre lake and is located on a circular dirt road. On the west and southwest sides of the loop, you will find 12 improved sites with water and power. The pads are simple hard-packed earth.

Twenty primitive sites line the north side of the loop. Again these are simple hard-packed earth pads. There are no tables, lantern posts, or grills here, so remember your camp stove. These sites are stacked side by side and lack privacy and elbowroom.

Facilities here are minimal at this time. In the campground there are two privies, one for men and one for women, and both have seen better days. There are no showers in the campground itself. You will have to either walk or drive around a lake slough to reach the main bathhouse at the park office, which is an original CCC structure. When I visited the campground for the book, a new bathhouse was being built next to the old building. In the meantime the current bathhouse is showing its age, but it does have hot showers and flush toilets.

Still, what the park lacks in facilities, it more than makes up for with its recreation and beauty. The longleaf pine forest mixed with a few hardwoods makes for a nice hike along one of the park's two trails—the Gazebo and the Bell. The 2-mile Bell Trail takes hikers across a scenic spillway formed by the dam that created the lake and around the banks of the lake itself. Once you reach the far end of either trail, be sure to look around for a nice view of the surrounding hillsides, something you don't normally see along the coast.

And I'd be remiss if I didn't mention the lake. Canoes and johnboats can be rented for $10 a day and paddleboats for $5 an hour. If you're a fisherman, the lake has bank fishing just off the Bell Trail or from a pier, or you can bring your own electric-powered boat. And during those hot, muggy days of summer, swimming in the lake provides a welcome respite from the heat. Just remember that this lake is a huge draw in the summer. The best time to visit is fall–spring.

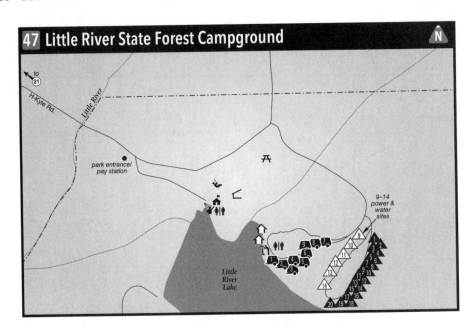

:: Getting There

From Atmore take AL 21 North 11 miles. The entrance is on the right.

GPS COORDINATES   N31° 37.211'   W87° 32.879'

48

Magnolia Branch Wildlife Reserve

"A little gem just outside of Atmore"

The story of the Poarch Band of Creek Indians is both tragic and a testament to perseverance. They are descendants of the original Creek Nation, which at one time populated most of Alabama and Georgia. For the most part the Creeks and federal government coexisted. In fact in 1790 a treaty was signed to develop an old American Indian trail into what would become a major trade route in the South, the Federal Road, which stretched from the Gulf of Mexico to north Georgia. The treaty allowed Creeks to establish businesses along the route to accommodate travelers. They built inns and served as guides and river pilots, and some became cattlemen, providing beef to the area.

Many travelers fell in love with the region and decided to settle the land, slowly forcing the Creeks out. Because of the rapid settlement, two factions of Creeks were formed who were at odds with one another, one friendly to the government and the other not. Tensions spilled over, and the two factions went to battle at the town of Burnt Corn.

:: Ratings

BEAUTY: ★ ★ ★ ★
PRIVACY: ★ ★
SPACIOUSNESS: ★ ★
QUIET: ★ ★ ★
SECURITY: ★ ★ ★ ★
CLEANLINESS: ★ ★ ★ ★

The Red Stick faction, which was hostile to the federal government, mounted a retaliatory attack on white settlers at Fort Mims, near present-day Bay Minette. The Creek Indian War, as it became known, finally ended with the Battle of Horseshoe Bend, which led to the forcible relocation of the American Indians to Oklahoma.

Some of the Creeks, however, were allowed to stay because of their wartime service to the U.S. government, but land was becoming scarce as timber companies began moving in and taking more and more land, and slowly the Creeks became impoverished.

It wasn't until the 1940s, with a lot of hard work and dedication, that the Poarch Band of Creek Indians started coming back. There were noticeable improvements to schools and in living conditions until finally in 1984 the federal government recognized the Poarch as an American Indian tribe, and almost 230,000 acres of land became their new reservation.

Today the Poarch Band of Creek Indians have overcome adversity and now own and operate Creek Indian Enterprises, a highly successful business venture pumping money into the reservation and local economy. The business runs casinos and this little gem just outside of Atmore, the Magnolia Branch Wildlife Preserve.

At the park you may encounter deer, raccoons, or any number of native species of wildlife. And keep your eyes to the sky for

:: Key Information

ADDRESS: 24 Big Creek Rd., Atmore, AL 36502

OPERATED BY: Creek Indian Enterprises

CONTACT: 251-446-3423; magnolia branch.com

OPEN: Year-round

SITES: 82

SITE AMENITIES: Picnic table, shared fire ring, water, power

ASSIGNMENT: First-come, first-serve or by reservation

REGISTRATION: Pay attendant at entrance or by reservation

FACILITIES: Flush toilets, hot showers, laundry, boat landing, playground, swimming, beach, volleyball court, horseshoe pit, zip line, fishing, camp store

PARKING: At each site

FEE: Improved (for up to 6 people), $20; primitive, $10 plus $1 per person

ELEVATION: 127'

RESTRICTIONS:

■ **Pets:** On leash only

■ **Fires:** In fire ring only

■ **Alcohol:** Prohibited

■ **Vehicles:** 2/site; sites A–M, 1/site with additional parking across the street near the restroom

■ **Other:** Quiet hours 10 p.m.–8 a.m.; 6 people/site

red-tailed hawks. The wetland area near the tent campground on Lake Menawah is beautiful with tall grass and the sound of water lapping on the shore.

With five water features and striking beaches, the park is obviously at its peak in the summer months as families from around the South come to swim in the wide creek and ponds, catch some rays on the beaches, fish in the lake, or maybe take a zip line across the water.

The main drawback for tent campers is the closeness of the campsites—you won't find much privacy and quietness, mainly in the summer months.

Tent campers will be sharing sites with RVers in sites 1–60. These sites, of course, include water and electricity. The sites have wide, gravel pull-through areas for easy RV access. Tent pads consist of gravel or narrow strips of dirt and grass off to the side of the sites. Sites 41–50 have little canopy for shade; towering pines provide shade for the other sites.

Sites 1–4, 15, 16, and 23–27 are waterfront sites; sites 1–4, 28, and 29 provide nice views of Rodeo Lake, while the remainder offer views and access to the beaches of Big Escambia Creek.

The nicest tent-only sites are sites A–O. These sites share a fire ring and have water and electricity. A single vehicle can park at each site, but the locations are close together, so be careful when you pull in. Parking is also available a few yards away across the camp road next to a restroom. The proximity of these sites to Lake Menawah grants you wonderful views and gorgeous sunsets. Sites O and N offer the best vistas, and site E is directly on the banks of the lake. Sites A, B, and C are on a pretty little finger of the lake.

A nice single-stall men's and women's restroom is across the main park road from the campground in the same area where you park. The fairly new, clean bathhouse is located in the RV area. It is spacious enough for the crowds who flock to the creek and lake

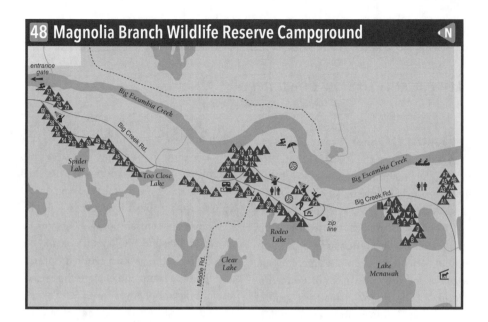

48 Magnolia Branch Wildlife Reserve Campground

in the summer. A coin-operated laundry is also available. It will take a slight trek or drive to get to the bathhouse, however. It's about 0.2 mile up the road from the tent campsites.

Unlimited primitive tent-camping opportunities are also available—simply pick your site. Remember, however, that *primitive* is the operative word for these sites—there are no amenities wherever you decide to pitch your tent. The only restriction on primitive campers is that they can't camp near the RV sites.

:: Getting There

From Atmore take AL 31 North 4.9 miles. Turn left onto North Canoe Road. Travel 3.4 miles and turn right onto Robinsonville Road. Travel 5.4 miles and turn right onto Big Creek Road. Travel 1.6 miles. The road comes to the entrance.

GPS COORDINATES   N31° 07.693'   W87° 22.293'

49

Meaher State Park

"Time seems to slow down here."

Granted, **Meaher State Park** is a small park in the Alabama State Park system, but magnificent sunsets and tranquil bayside camping make up for what it lacks in size.

Now let me preface this description by saying that if you are looking for a campground with plenty of on-site amenities and activities for kids, this may not be the one to choose. Oh, there's a small playground, but as for activities within, your kids will be left wanting. Meaher State Park doesn't have all of the trappings of many of the Alabama state parks. You won't find horseback riding, hiking trails, or lake swimming. What you will find is a place to just kick back and relax. Time seems to slow down here.

Meaher State Park sits right on Mobile Bay, just south of the second-largest river delta in the country, the Mobile–Tensaw Delta. Five rivers join together here, funneling runoff from several Southeastern states into the Gulf of Mexico to form one of the richest ecological areas on the coast. While at the park you'll be treated to the sight of the once-endangered brown pelican soaring high and then crashing into the water to catch its daily meals. You may also see large herons—some big enough to cast a huge shadow as they pass over—soaring high overhead, or maybe, just maybe, you'll catch a glimpse of an alligator or two.

Meaher is centrally located between the city of Mobile and the bay's Eastern Shore, which makes the park an excellent location to pitch base camp and explore the region's fascinating 300-plus-year history.

Start first by crossing the causeway to pay a visit to the Five Rivers Delta Resource Center. The center is operated by the Alabama Department of Conservation and Natural Resources and admission is free. Take a walk through the exhibit hall to see the many different species of wildlife that call the delta home, and then take in a movie in the center's theater. Simply ask one of the staff about the available nature documentaries, and they'll plug one in for you. And while you're there, take a cruise with Delta Safaris, which offers daytime 2-hour cruises of the delta and special Gators after Dark trips. If you want to see an alligator, you will!

To the west is the city of Mobile, Alabama's port city. Mobile is known as the "Mother of Mystics" because it is the birthplace of Mardi Gras in the United States. Unlike the New Orleans version, Mobile's version is family-friendly but still a good time, with plenty of beads and MoonPies, which are tossed to parade-goers.

If you like shopping, then head over to the Eastern Shore towns of Spanish Fort, Daphne, and Fairhope for a wide range of

:: Ratings

BEAUTY: ★ ★ ★ ★
PRIVACY: ★ ★ ★ ★
SPACIOUSNESS: ★ ★ ★
QUIET: ★ ★ ★
SECURITY: ★ ★ ★ ★
CLEANLINESS: ★ ★ ★ ★

:: Key Information

ADDRESS: 5200 Battleship Pkwy. E., Spanish Fort, AL 36527

OPERATED BY: Alabama State Parks

CONTACT: 251-626-5529; alapark.com/meaher

OPEN: Year-round

SITES: 56

SITE AMENITIES: Picnic table, grill, water, power

ASSIGNMENT: First-come, first-serve

REGISTRATION: Pay attendant at entrance

FACILITIES: Flush toilets, hot showers, laundry, playground, fishing pier

PARKING: At each site

FEE: $30

ELEVATION: 6'

RESTRICTIONS:
- **Pets:** On leash only
- **Fires:** In grill only
- **Alcohol:** Prohibited
- **Vehicles:** 2/site
- **Other:** Quiet hours 10 p.m.–6 a.m.; 1 tent (4 people)/site

stores, as well as an equally wide range of annual festivals.

Meaher State Park is on the main highway, the causeway (US 90) that connects the two sides of the bay. That close proximity can sometimes mean that traffic sounds will invade your peace and quiet, but come late afternoon and evening, things die down to a whisper.

Every site provides an excellent bay view, with shrimp and recreational boats plying the waters and cargo ships and barges heading to the Gulf of Mexico. My favorites are sites 43 and 44, which sit right on the bay, are more secluded, and are farther away from the highway than the other sites. Each site has water, electricity, a picnic table, and a grill. Tent sites are simple grass areas near each site's paved parking area.

The bathhouses are modern and immaculate with hot showers, flush toilets, and a laundry. And security is excellent as well, with a chain-link gate that's locked after-hours. Campers receive a code to enter and leave, and a camp host is always present at site 38.

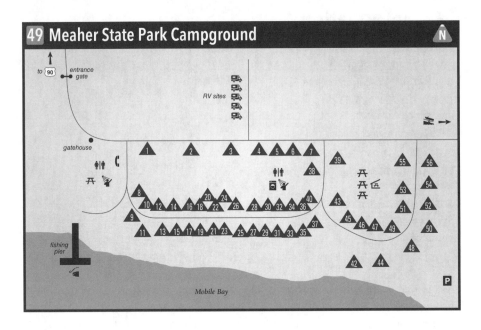

:: Getting There

From Mobile take US 90 East 6.5 miles. The entrance is on the right.

GPS COORDINATES   N30° 40.174'   W87° 56.153'

50

Old St. Stephens Historical Park

"Old St. Stephens features a 100-acre clear-blue lake rimmed with beautiful white limestone bluffs."

Old St. Stephens Historical Park is unique in that it is an active research site. Students from the University of South Alabama and volunteers from around the region spend months with spade in hand, piecing together the history of this 220-year-old city.

In a span of 30 years, Old St. Stephens saw Spanish and American forts and served as the territorial capital of Alabama.

The Spanish governor of Mobile, Juan Vicente Folch, built the original fort at Old St. Stephens in 1789. He realized that this location, high atop a steep limestone bluff on the banks of the Tombigbee River, was perfect for a settlement because boats heading north on the river would be forced to land there as the river began to get more shallow. The fort was turned over to the United States in 1799 and began growing. In its heyday the town sported high-class boarding houses, hotels, theaters, and Alabama's first chartered school, Washington Academy.

:: Ratings

> **BEAUTY:** ★ ★ ★ ★
> **PRIVACY:** ★ ★ ★
> **SPACIOUSNESS:** ★ ★
> **QUIET:** ★ ★ ★
> **SECURITY:** ★ ★ ★
> **CLEANLINESS:** ★ ★ ★ ★

In 1817 the Alabama Territory was formed and Old St. Stephens became the state's capital, which explains the park's motto, "where Alabama began." But in one year the capital was moved to Cahawba, and with it, the population moved, too, mostly relocating a few miles away to New St. Stephens.

The town quickly went into decline and was reclaimed by nature, but today through the efforts of the university's archeological department and many volunteers, you can walk the streets of the long-forgotten town along a 0.8-mile-long trail that takes you back in time. As you pass through the redbud and dogwood trees, interpretive signs tell the story of life in the town that once boasted more than 7,000 residents. Street signs mark the intersections of main thoroughfares, and white posts indicate the property lines of residential homes, banks, and hotels. Many house numbers are identified along the route.

As you make your way to the end of the hike, you will come to one of the town's finest hotels, the Globe. This is where the main dig is currently underway. You will see the building foundation as well as the work the archeologists are doing.

But Old St. Stephens isn't only about history. It's also about nature. The site features a 100-acre clear-blue lake rimmed with beautiful white limestone bluffs.

:: Key Information

ADDRESS: 1176 Old St. Stephens Rd., St. Stephens, AL 36569	**REGISTRATION:** Pay attendant at camp store or by phone
OPERATED BY: Old St. Stephens Historical Commission	**FACILITIES:** Flush toilets, hot showers, camp store
CONTACT: 251-247-2622; oldststephens.com	**PARKING:** At each site
OPEN: Year-round	**FEE:** $10
SITES: 34	**ELEVATION:** 103'
SITE AMENITIES: Lakeview Campground–Picnic table, fire ring, grill, water, power; Cedar Ridge Campground–Picnic table, fire ring, water, power	**RESTRICTIONS:**
	■ **Pets:** On leash only
	■ **Fires:** In fire ring or grill only
	■ **Alcohol:** Prohibited
ASSIGNMENT: First-come, first-serve or by reservation	■ **Vehicles:** 2/site
	■ **Other:** Quiet hours 10 p.m.–6 a.m.

There are plenty of opportunities to take a walk and catch a scenic lake view from atop these bluffs, or enjoy a lakeside view of the bluffs themselves.

Between the two campgrounds you'll find beautiful wetlands with an array of colorful wildflowers and butterflies. With the bluffs as a backdrop, this is a photographer's paradise.

And then there is the Tombigbee River, the reason that Old St. Stephens came into existence in the first place. From a landing you can watch the wide, green river meander by.

This is one of the few historical parks in Alabama that is not operated by the Alabama Historic Commission. Instead, the Old St. Stephens Historical Commission is charged with maintaining the facility. As with many historic sites, Old St. Stephens is facing a financial crisis and is seeing its budget cut drastically; dedicated volunteers do a remarkable job of keeping the park operating.

The park has two campgrounds. The first, Lakeview, sits on a limestone bluff high above the lake. The highlight is the view of the lake, with its deep-blue water. The best sites are 5, 7, 9, and 11. These are right at the bluff edge, so it's imperative that you be safe and keep clear of the drop-off, especially if you're camping with kids. The two sites to avoid if you can are 17 and 18, which are on the edge of the campground road.

All sites in the Lakeview Campground have fire rings, picnic tables, water, power, and grills. You'll also find a very nice bathhouse with showers, toilets, and plenty of room.

The second campground, Cedar Ridge, is a straight line of campsites that are advertised as primitive but are far from that—with fire rings, picnic tables, water, and power. The sites are a bit close together but nothing that will be distracting from the park's tranquility. There is no bathhouse here, but there is easy access to the lake for swimming. Be warned: It is a deep lake and no lifeguards are on duty, so be safe.

As you drive between the two campgrounds, you will pass a small camp store that stocks basic necessities.

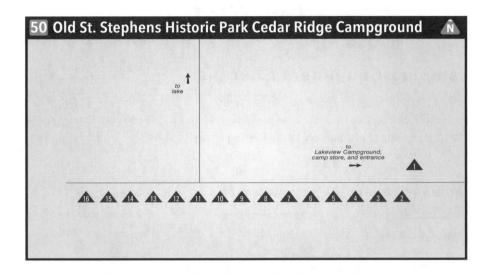

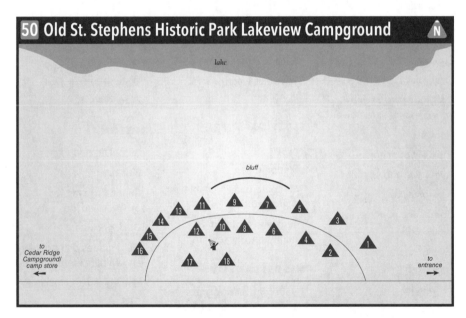

:: Getting There

From Jackson take US 43/AL 13 3.3 miles. Turn right onto County Road 34. Travel 6.3 miles. Make a slight right onto Howell Road (look for the park sign in the middle of the fork pointing to the right). Travel 0.1 mile and make another slight right onto Cement Plant Road. Travel 0.6 mile, and the entrance and park office are on the right. The first campground, Lakeview, is an additional 2 miles past the office.

GPS COORDINATES   N31° 33.503'   W88° 02.480'

APPENDIX A

● ●

Camping-Equipment Checklist

I keep a plastic storage container full of the essentials for car camping, except for the large and bulky items on this list, so they're ready to go when I am. It's essential that you make a last-minute check of the inventor and resupply anything that's low or missing—then away you go.

COOKING UTENSILS

Bottle opener

Bottles of salt, pepper, spices, sugar, and cooking oil and maple syrup in waterproof, spillproof containers

Can opener

Corkscrew

Cups, plastic or tin

Dish soap *(biodegradable)*, sponge, and towel

Flatware

Food of your choice

Frying pan and spatula

Fuel for stove

Lighter and matches in waterproof container

Plates

Pocketknife

Pot with lid

Stove

Tin foil

Wooden spoon

FIRST-AID KIT

Adhesive bandages

Aspirin

First-aid cream

Gauze pads

Insect repellent

Moleskin

Sunscreen/lip balm

Tape and waterproof adhesive

SLEEP GEAR

Pillow

Sleeping bag

Sleeping pad, inflatable or insulated

Tent with ground tarp, rainfly, and stakes

MISCELLANEOUS

Bath soap *(biodegradable)*, washcloth, and towel

Camp chair

Candles

Cooler

Duct tape

Flashlight/headlamp

Hammer

Nylon rope

Paper towels

Plastic zip-top bags

Sunglasses

Toilet paper

Water bottle

Wool blanket

OPTIONAL

Barbecue grill

Binoculars

Canoe or kayak with paddles and life vests

Deck of cards

Field guides on bird, plant, and wildlife identification

Fishing rod and tackle

GPS unit

Lantern

Maps *(road, trail, topographic, and so on)*

APPENDIX B

• •

Sources of Information

The following is a partial list of agencies, associations, and organizations to write or call for information on outdoor-recreation opportunities in Alabama.

ALABAMA TOURISM DEPARTMENT
alabama.travel
401 Adams Ave., Ste. 126
P.O. Box 4927
Montgomery, AL 36103-4927
(800) 252-2272

ALABAMA DEPARTMENT OF CONSERVATION AND NATURAL RESOURCES
outdooralabama.com
64 N. Union St.
Montgomery, AL 36130
(334) 242-3486

ALABAMA DEPARTMENT OF ECONOMIC AND COMMUNITY AFFAIRS
RECREATION AND CONSERVATION UNIT
adeca.alabama.gov
P.O. Box 5690
Montgomery, AL 36103
(334) 242-5100

ALABAMA FORESTRY COMMISSION
forestry.state.al.us
513 Madison Ave.
Montgomery, AL 36104
(334) 240-9300

ALABAMA HISTORIC COMMISSION
preserve.ala.org
468 S. Perry St.
Montgomery, AL 36104
(334) 242-3184

ALABAMA MOUNTAIN LAKES TOURIST ASSOCIATION
northalabama.org
402 Sherman St.

P.O. Box 2537
Decatur, AL 35602
(800) 648-5381

ALABAMA STATE PARKS
alapark.com
64 N. Union St.
Montgomery, AL 36130
(800) 252-7275

SHOALS ENVIRONMENTAL ALLIANCE
sea.tinywebs.org
P.O. Box 699
Sheffield, AL 35660

TENNESSEE VALLEY AUTHORITY
tva.com/river/recreation/camping.htm
400 W. Summit Hill Dr., WT 11A
Knoxville, TN 37902

US ARMY CORPS OF ENGINEERS
www.sam.usace.army.mil
109 Saint Joseph St.
Mobile, AL 36602

US FOREST SERVICE
fs.usda.gov/alabama
2946 Chestnut St.
Montgomery, AL 36107
(334) 832-4470

WILDSOUTH
wildsouth.org
11312 AL 33, Ste. 1
Moulton, AL 35650

INDEX

● ●

ABOUT THE AUTHOR

Joe Cuhaj hails from Mahwah, New Jersey, and despite what you may think about the Garden State—ignore what you've seen on *Jersey Shore*—this is where his love of hiking and camping began. Living in the shadow of New York's Harriman–Bear Mountain State Park, where the first section of the Appalachian Trail was built, and atop a foothill of the Appalachian Mountains, Joe and his high school friends would take to the woods at any opportunity for camping, hiking, and canoeing.

After graduating and spending four years in the U.S. Navy as a radioman, Joe moved to Mobile, Alabama, in 1980 with his wife, Maggie, a native of the area, and he immediately fell in love with the state's amazing environmental diversity and recreational opportunities. Since then he's explored much of Alabama by foot over its hundreds of miles of hiking trails and by water along its myriad rivers and coastal waterways, taking the time to enjoy the state's many campgrounds along the way.

As a freelance writer, Joe was afforded the opportunity to share these adventures with readers in two books, *Hiking Alabama* and *Paddling Alabama* (Falcon Books). He has also coauthored a book on another favorite pastime of his, titled *Baseball in Mobile* (Arcadia Publishing), about the history of the sport in the Port City.

Besides being a writer, Joe worked many years in radio as a news reporter and anchor, sports commentator, music director, and program director before becoming a software programmer. In 2006 he was honored with the Southern Volunteer of the Year Award, presented by the American Hiking Society for his work in building hiking trails throughout the state and promoting hiking and the environment with the nonprofit Alabama Hiking Trail Society.

Joe and Maggie live in Daphne, on the Eastern Shore of Mobile Bay. They are the proud parents of one daughter, Kellie, and have two grandchildren, Cora and Steven.

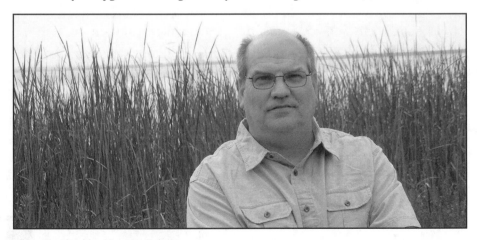

photographed by Maggie Cuhaj

DEAR CUSTOMERS AND FRIENDS,

SUPPORTING YOUR INTEREST IN OUTDOOR ADVENTURE, travel, and an active lifestyle is central to our operations, from the authors we choose to the locations we detail to the way we design our books. Menasha Ridge Press was incorporated in 1982 by a group of veteran outdoorsmen and professional outfitters. For 25 years now, we've specialized in creating books that benefit the outdoors enthusiast.

Almost immediately, Menasha Ridge Press earned a reputation for revolutionizing outdoors- and travel-guidebook publishing. For such activities as canoeing, kayaking, hiking, backpacking, and mountain biking, we established new standards of quality that transformed the whole genre, resulting in outdoor-recreation guides of great sophistication and solid content. Menasha Ridge continues to be outdoor publishing's greatest innovator.

The folks at Menasha Ridge Press are as at home on a white-water river or mountain trail as they are editing a manuscript. The books we build for you are the best they can be, because we're responding to your needs. Plus, we use and depend on them ourselves.

We look forward to seeing you on the river or the trail. If you'd like to contact us directly, join in at www.trekalong.com or visit us at www.menasharidge.com. We thank you for your interest in our books and the natural world around us all.

SAFE TRAVELS,

Bob Sehlinger

BOB SEHLINGER
PUBLISHER